Praise for *The Nurse's Reality Shift*

"Neal-Boylan's book, impressive in its scope, is a call to action. She clearly illustrates how the problems of today ARE the same problems we grappled with 50 years ago. She calls on us to act in an integrated, meaningful way to implement decisions made decades ago and make changes necessary to ensure the future of nursing practice and nursing education."

–Sharron E. Guillett, PhD, RN
State Director, Nursing Programs
Stratford University, Falls Church, Virginia

"An inspiring nursing leader, Neal-Boylan provides a compelling critique of the current state of the science and art of nursing through a lens of the past and present. She challenges readers to retain that lens to envision the future of the profession. This book is a must-read for all nurse clinicians, academicians, and researchers."

–Maryanne Davidson, DNSc, APRN, CPNP
Associate Professor of Nursing
Sacred Heart University School of Nursing

"This book is a highly realistic view of where nursing care and nursing education were in the past and where they are now; it is also a thought-provoking discussion for all who strive to educate and train nurses for the future. Nurses educated to prepare future nurses must retain their nursing skills to produce nurses who are qualified graduates. Included is advice for each of us to take care of ourselves to be able to care for others. The author reminds us that nurses are made, not born. I recommend this wonderful book to everyone who considers becoming a caregiver."

–Shirley A. Patterson, MSN
U.S. Army Nurse Corps, Retired

The Nurse's Reality Shift

Using History to Transform the Future

Leslie Neal-Boylan,
PhD, CRRN, APRN-BC, FNP, FAAN

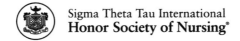

Sigma Theta Tau International
Honor Society of Nursing®

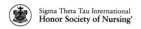
Sigma Theta Tau International
Honor Society of Nursing®

> The Honor Society of Nursing, Sigma Theta Tau International (STTI) is a nonprofit organization founded in 1922 whose mission is to support the learning, knowledge, and professional development of nurses committed to making a difference in health worldwide. Members include practicing nurses, instructors, researchers, policymakers, entrepreneurs and others. STTI's 496 chapters are located at 678 institutions of higher education throughout Australia, Botswana, Brazil, Canada, Colombia, Ghana, Hong Kong, Japan, Kenya, Malawi, Mexico, the Netherlands, Pakistan, Portugal, Singapore, South Africa, South Korea, Swaziland, Sweden, Taiwan, Tanzania, United Kingdom, United States, and Wales. More information about STTI can be found online at www.nursingsociety.org.

Sigma Theta Tau International
550 West North Street
Indianapolis, IN, USA 46202

To order additional books, buy in bulk, or order for corporate use, contact Nursing Knowledge International at 888.NKI.4YOU (888.654.4968/US and Canada) or +1.317.634.8171 (outside US and Canada).

To request a review copy for course adoption, email solutions@nursingknowledge.org or call 888. NKI.4YOU (888.654.4968/US and Canada) or +1.317.634.8171 (outside US and Canada).

To request author information, or for speaker or other media requests, contact Marketing, Honor Society of Nursing, Sigma Theta Tau International at 888.634.7575 (US and Canada) or +1.317.634.8171 (outside US and Canada).

ISBN: 9781938835629
EPUB ISBN: 9781938835636
PDF ISBN: 9781938835643
MOBI ISBN: 9781938835650

Library of Congress Cataloging-in-Publication Data

Neal-Boylan, Leslie, author.
The nurse's reality shift : using history to transform the future / Leslie Neal-Boylan.
  p. ; cm.
Includes bibliographical references.
ISBN 978-1-938835-62-9 (print : alk. paper) -- ISBN 978-1-938835-63-6 (EPUB) -- ISBN 978-1-938835-64-3 (PDF) -- ISBN 978-1-938835-65-0 (MOBI)
I. Sigma Theta Tau International, issuing body. II. Title.
[DNLM: 1. Nursing--trends--United States. 2. Education, Nursing--United States. 3. History of Nursing--United States. 4. History, 20th Century--United States. WY 16 AA1]
RT42
610.73--dc23
                    2014038672

Antique stethoscope copyright and courtesy of Douglas Arbittier, MD, MBA, www.medicalantiques.com.

First Printing, 2014

Publisher: Dustin Sullivan
Acquisitions Editor: Emily Hatch
Editorial Coordinator: Paula Jeffers
Cover Designer: Rebecca Batchelor
Indexer: Joy Dean Lee

Principal Book Editor: Carla Hall
Development and Project Editor: Kate Shoup
Proofreader: Barbara Bennett
Interior Design/Page Layout: Katy Bodenmiller

Dedication

For my father, Edward Rotkoff (may his memory be for a blessing), who loved and respected nurses and whom I miss every day.

Also, for three sisters, Anne Marie Boylan, RN, Margaret Boyle, RN, and Bridget Boylan, RN. They were three Irish nurses who struggled through discrimination as students and young nurses to make wonderful contributions to nursing.

My sincere thanks to all of the nurses who took the time to respond to the survey. Thank you for all that you do.

Acknowledgments

To Claryn Spies, BA, with many thanks for her time, effort, and invaluable contributions to this book. Thank you so much to the wonderful editorial staff at STTI Publishing, especially Emily Hatch, Kate Shoup, and Carla Hall.

About the Author

Leslie Neal-Boylan, PhD, CRRN, APRN-BC, FNP, FAAN, is associate dean and professor at Quinnipiac University in Hamden, Connecticut. She earned her BSN from Rutgers University, her MSN from San Jose State University, and her PhD in nursing from George Mason University. She received a post-master's certificate as a family nurse practitioner (FNP) from Marymount University. She is a board-certified family nurse practitioner and is certified in rehabilitation nursing, home health nursing, and rheumatology. She maintains a clinical practice as an FNP. Neal-Boylan has maintained a clinical practice for 30 years including the last 15 years, during which she has worked in academe full time. She has authored and/or edited almost 100 peer-reviewed publications, including eight books. Her research focus has been on the nursing workforce, most recently concerning registered nurses with disabilities. However, she has also published on topics related to geriatric patient care, the nurse practitioner role, and chronic illness.

Table of Contents

Introduction

Those who cannot remember the past are condemned to repeat it.

−George Santayana

Presumably, since you are reading this book, either you are a nurse or you want to be one. Let me speak to you, then, as a colleague and a confidante. As nurses, we have much to be proud of. Nevertheless, if we take an objective view, it is clear that in many ways, we have not come as far in the nursing profession as our forebears intended. Like any large family, we have skeletons in our closet, and we don't like to air our dirty laundry. But if we are to progress as a profession, it's time we deal with both. The sad fact is, many of the problems we face as nurses today have existed since our beginning. If we want to have any hope of solving them, we must first acknowledge them.

This book is not intended to be a history book. Many others have written our history far better than I ever could. Rather, it is a look back at how far we've come while spotlighting issues and events that continue to plague us.

The first part of this book delves into significant events in nursing's history from 1900 to 1970. In this part, you will learn the origin of some of nursing's ongoing concerns. No doubt, you will find it interesting to read the words of early nurse leaders as they lament issues still very familiar to us.

The second part of the book features survey responses of real live nurses of today. These nurses, who come from various educational levels and work settings throughout the United States, range in age from 23 years to 73 years. Both female and male nurses responded. Although most were Caucasian, there was a mix of Hispanic, Asian, African-American, and Native-American nurses. They span all educational levels of RNs from associate degree and diploma through the doctorate. (That's why some of their suggestions contradict others. It's a matter of perspective!) A total of 608 nurses responded to the survey. While the survey was approved by the Quinnipiac University institutional review board, it was not intended to be a research study. Rather, it was meant to provide information to supplement the literature and to further enlighten us about the pressing issues of the day. Rarely did a nurse respond to all the open-ended questions. Most seemed to pick and choose, so my attempts to aggregate the data were not helpful. Nonetheless, several themes resonated with everyone.

The third part of this book uses the literature and my own observations over the past 35 years in nursing to look into what could be if we were to learn from our past. As you read, listen to the voices of our nursing forebears and of your contemporaries. Are their voices reflective of your own voice? If nothing else, I hope this book stirs dialogue among us.

Each chapter begins with a story. Most of these were written by my mother, Natalie Rotkoff, whose nursing career began in 1953, about her experiences or those of her mother, who became a nurse in the 1920s. I think the stories inject a bit of reality and humor. Coming from my own family makes them special to me, and I hope you will enjoy them. I'm sure you can relate to them no matter how old you are. After all, while the profession may have changed in some ways and stagnated in others, nurses share the common experience of being nurses and having a passion for this most special profession.

So, please join me now as we take a no-holds-barred look at where we've been and where we can go if we let go of some of our prejudices and preconceptions. I'd love to hear your opinions and thoughts after you do. Thanks for taking the time to read this book. I know how busy you are!

Leslie Neal-Boylan

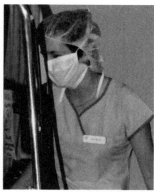

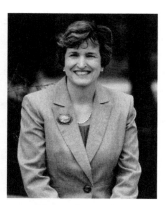

The author as a young obstetrics nurse.

The author, 2013.

Inspiration

Rose Fierstein Lebowitz, my grandmother ("As Probie, 1918"), was born in 1900 and graduated from the Cleveland Hospital School of Nursing in the early 1920s. She was a Hungarian immigrant and became a nurse when Jewish women were discouraged from such work. She often worked in the emergency room but also cared for family and neighbors in need.

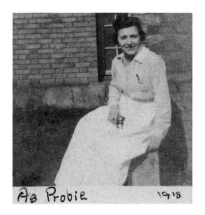

As Probie   1918

Natalie Joy Lebowitz Rotkoff, my mother, was born in 1933 and graduated in 1953 from the nursing school associated with Brooklyn Jewish Hospital in Brooklyn, New York. In the bottom photo, she is pictured (far left) with two other nursing students, one of whom became a lifelong friend. My mother took time off from nursing while my brothers and I were growing up but, informally, she took care of family and friends and sometimes perfect strangers who needed help. She worked as a school nurse and in a veterans hospital, and was the assistant director of nursing in a large nursing home. I was always amazed at her diagnostic acumen and her memory for things she had learned many years before. She taught me why nursing is so vital to the health and survival of humanity.

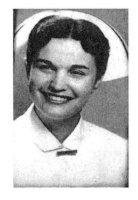

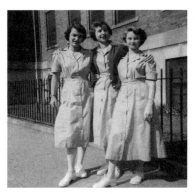

Chapter 1
Nurses Are Made, Not Born: Educational Reform Frames the Profession (1900–1935)

My grandmother graduated as a registered nurse in 1920. My mother remembers her as the breadwinner, although it was unusual for a mother to work outside the home at that time. My mother remembers a phone in the house provided by AT&T because my grandmother was a nurse and others might need to reach her. Friends and neighbors partook of this and my grandmother always complied, occasionally bringing my mother along when she went next door or across the street to tend to an ailing neighbor. My mother, who would go on rounds with my grandmother, remembers hysteria related to WWII because of sons away fighting, food rationing, and domestic concerns in single parent homes. After visiting a neighbor once, my mother asked, "That woman is such a neurotic. How do you stand it?" My grandmother, instilled with respect for confidentiality around her patient's troubles, would never reply. My mother clearly remembers the relief that would appear on the faces of dying neighbors when they saw my grandmother arrive, taking comfort from her "beautiful countenance and professional demeanor" as she assisted them to die at home.

The first few decades of the 20th century were highly significant in establishing a framework for the nascent profession of nursing. During this period, nursing leaders proposed many changes in education and practice that set the stage for the future. Much of what arose from their discussions resonates today, as many of the issues confronting them remain with us in some form or fashion. It is fascinating to read about the presentations and discussions that took place as nursing struggled to define itself and differentiate itself from layperson caregiving.

Not Everyone Can Be a Nurse

Prior to the opening of nurse training schools in 1873, anyone could consider oneself to be a nurse. When formal training began, it became vital to establish standards and guidelines to move nursing from the public image of the family caretaker to one of a trained professional. In 1893, nursing leaders met to form the Association of Superintendents of Training Schools for Nurses—later the National League for Nursing—and develop its bylaws. One of the requirements for membership in the association was graduation from a training school that provided at least 2 years of formal instruction. The training school superintendents who comprised the membership of the Association of Superintendents of Training Schools for Nurses believed that not everyone could be a nurse. Admission criteria were created, but were altered as the need for nurses rose and fell. There was significant variability in admission requirements. Interestingly, the public remains confused about just who is a nurse. As will become clear in this book, the profession is largely to blame.

The superintendents also faced the challenge of weighing theory and practice, a debate that continues to this day. For much of the 20th century, the connection between training schools and hospitals has influenced this discussion.

A Focus on Critical Thinking

Today, nurse educators talk about the need to instill critical thinking as a relatively new concept. However, a focus of nursing education has always been to teach students to think for themselves. As one nurse leader stated in 1915 (Gillette, as cited in Birnbach & Lewenson, 1991, p. 39):

> We must teach [the student] that ready acceptance of everything she finds in print shows a lack of thought.... She should be taught to verify statements by looking them up in some book of recognized authority. She should be taught to consider the author and the date of publication, and to ask, "Will it work?"

Are today's nursing students taught to verify information, to analyze the articles they read, and to question the source and the author's motivation? I don't think this occurs enough. Nursing students may be taught to analyze a patient case and to propose ideas for management, but most are not encouraged to read broadly and to bring knowledge of literature and the world to their discussions. We continue to talk about the public image of nursing and lament that there are still people who consider it a vocation rather than a profession. However, while we require classes in the liberal arts, do we ask students to bring that learning to bear when they examine issues related to nursing?

Once the profession began to speak of and develop guidelines for uniformity, nurse leaders recommended a standard entrance exam—"thorough English education and a knowledge of literature, and matters of general interest" (Snively, as cited in Birnbach & Lewenson, 1991, p. 12)—as well as a uniform length of education composed of exposure to specific clinical areas. Interestingly, knowledge of English and literature were deemed necessary "for those who minister to the sick" (Snively, as cited in Birnbach & Lewenson, 1991, p. 12). Today, it has become increasingly apparent that nursing students (as well as students of other disciplines) are often poorly prepared to speak and write English even if they are native born. The inability to write well often stems from a lack of exposure to good writing, namely literature. Today's society has placed less emphasis on reading anything, let alone literature, than on watching reality TV, using technology, or playing video games. Furthermore, students today do not typically possess a breadth of knowledge in areas "of general interest."

This has most likely hampered the nursing profession as we have sought over the decades to be viewed as scholars and professionals. If one has little awareness of world or societal events and is not well-spoken or well-read, it is hard to expect that one will be taken seriously. Early nurse leaders felt that students should be "independent searchers for knowledge" (Gillette, as cited in Birnbach & Lewenson, 1991, p. 37) and should receive instruction in the use of the library and the importance of keeping current with nursing *and* medical journals. Another nurse leader quoted an unknown source, saying "We wish that the pupil be treated as one who intends, and who is expected to learn for himself, rather than as one who is to be supplied with knowledge by us out of the stores of our information" (Harmer, as cited in Birnbach & Lewenson, 1991, p. 50). Nonetheless, in the nursing classrooms of today, we see faculty more concerned with "nurturing" students than with maintaining high expectations for student performance. This may be due in part to the reluctance to fail students in classes because of tuition-driven requirements, but it may also be due to the gradual lowering of the standards for writing, reading, and exam performance.

I think we are more demanding with regard to clinical and skills performance than we are in the classroom. We recognize that students must be safe practitioners, so we require strict adherence to each step of, for example, putting in a catheter. This is necessary. However, if we don't maintain the same high standard in the classroom, can we blame others for continuing to see us as technicians rather than as critical thinkers? Also, the necessity to complete each and every skill with precision precludes admitting students who may be excellent thinkers but have physical disabilities that prevent them from performing a technical task without help. Does a good nurse have to be able to perform each and every skill independently and "the way it has always been done"? Can we acknowledge that a nurse with a good brain can direct others to perform tasks that he or she is unable to perform himself or herself?

Clinical Experience

Another issue that is as relevant today as it was early in the 20th century is that of clinical time. How much is enough? Too much? Is it being used appropriately? Hospital experience was thought to be integral to nurse training, and superintendants took great pains to ensure that students received intensive experiences in a variety of areas. It was recognized early that nursing students required an education that exposed them to a variety of specialty areas, but that curricula would benefit from uniformity among schools.

Schools of nursing continue to debate how much clinical time and what types of experiences really are necessary. Outside forces such as the decline in the willingness of some hospitals to take on students and restrictions on exposure of patients to endless streams of students from a variety of healthcare disciplines have affected how much clinical time students actually receive. Many schools have responded by purchasing expensive simulation equipment and supplementing clinical experience with real patients by using mannequins and computer technology. In addition, schools have hit upon creative solutions by finding clinical experiences outside the hospital setting. This makes sense, given that most patients are now cared for in community and outpatient settings. Still, nursing students, regardless of their type of training program, lament that they have insufficient clinical experience. Rarely do they feel well-prepared when they graduate to assume their clinical responsibilities (Neal-Boylan, 2013).

Early nurse leaders also spoke to the necessity of faculty remaining involved in clinical practice. They recognized that a nurse's first duty is to his or her patients. Further, they foresaw that nurse administrators—whether in schools of nursing or in hospital settings—should have specialized training to carry out their responsibilities (Taylor, as cited in Birnbach & Lewenson, 1991, p. 61). Currently, one does not require an advanced degree to become an administrator, nor are faculty required to maintain clinical currency. How can we teach students if we are not "walking the walk"?

Many faculty consider continuing education seminars and conferences worthy substitutes for engaging in clinical practice. This appears contradictory to what we tell our students—that you cannot just hear or read about patient care to be able to practice it competently. Others say that being a clinical educator is sufficient to keep one current. Clearly, the instructor must know what is appropriate on a given unit in order to teach it effectively. But is that the same as managing one's own patient load or delivering care for which one is completely responsible? Whether weekly or only during the summer or holiday time, it is important that nursing faculty engage clinically as direct care providers.

Early nurse leaders were strong proponents of what we would now call a "nurse residency." They believed that if a nursing student wanted to be prepared to take on a hospital position or a position as a superintendent or faculty in a school of nursing after graduation and certification, that student should spend some time in the final year of school learning how to be an administrator. The third or final year of school was considered to be the period in which the student could begin to assimilate what he or she had learned. Even early in the 20th century, nurse graduates were remarking that they wished they had had another year of school in which to become more proficient in all areas of clinical practice.

This is an issue that may never be resolved—at least not until such time that the entire way in which we educate nurses is changed. Professional nurses must know theory: the whys and wherefores behind the care we provide. But they also need actual hands-on experience, only some of which can be gained using high-fidelity mannequins. Should baccalaureate education be a 5-year program with the last year being a supervised residency? Is a one-semester capstone sufficient to acclimate the graduating student to the reality of nursing?

Physicians Feel Threatened

As nurse training formalized, with an emphasis on learning the science of disease and treatment, physicians began to feel threatened. In 1999, Ruby stated that "institutional oppression and control over nursing practice continues to be a reality despite increased numbers of women physicians" (Ruby, 1999, p. 25). Some 15 years later, this continues, despite a recent upsurge in conversation about interprofessionalism. Interdisciplinary teamwork has been a focus of clinical nursing practice for decades. Recently, however, physicians have recognized the value of interprofessionalism and are trying to integrate it into medical education. Unfortunately, this process has a long way to go. While the word "interprofessional" is used, it is clearly misunderstood, as physicians continue to talk about the "medical community" and claim they represent the voices of all healthcare professionals.

Lateral Violence

Lately, there has been much mention in the literature about lateral violence, or the verbal abuse or neglect of nursing students and new nurses. History does truly repeat itself, and this is but one example. Early in nursing education, fear and awe were the motivators in nursing education. There was a lot of attrition in nurse training programs, in large part because the lives of the students were closely governed and the demands were great. By 1932, nurse leaders were talking about changing this paradigm (Hodgkins, as cited in Birnbach & Lewenson, 1991).

Community Nursing

Nursing has always prided itself on being holistic—looking at the entire individual with regard to mental, social, and physical health—and prevention. Presentations from early in the 20th century proclaimed that it was the nurse who was in large part responsible for the success of many efforts to eradicate disease. This was because the nurse was in a position to identify the societal factors that affect the disease and work with patients within the community setting to minimize their effects. Public and community health education were considered important in nursing education for this reason (Tucker, as cited in Birnbach & Lewenson, 1991). Today, nurses educate patients about preventive practices regardless of the setting, but there is a resurgence of interest in caring for patients in the community as fewer patients are hospitalized for less time.

Historically, patients did not want to go to hospitals because they were places of filth, contagion, and strict rules and regulations, mostly from nurses. Before nursing education and care became more standardized, untrained people provided care that was sporadic and inadequate. Most people were cared for at home by family caregivers, typically widowed or spinster females. Later, these "nurses" were hired to provide care (Reverby, 1987). Most patients today go to the hospital only for surgery or serious illness. Fortunately, the standards for cleanliness and care have improved significantly. However, most nursing schools still provide most of their clinical teaching in hospitals and emphasize acute care nursing. Community health education typically occurs in one course in which students get clinical exposure to home and public health nursing.

Public health nursing, which began in the 1800s, grew during the 20th century despite uncertainty about the actual role of the public health nurse (Reverby, 1987). Overall, public health nurses liked their jobs and often received better pay than their colleagues in hospitals. Just like today, this type of nursing allowed nurses to be far more autonomous and independent than in other settings. Public health agencies valued a strong academic education, including nursing theory. And while public health was the smallest practice area, it was considered the most elite by nurses. Before physicians organized restrictions of autonomous nursing practice in public health settings, nurses were without physician supervision and could treat and educate underserved communities (Ruby, 1999).

Similar to today, "nursing could...lead to very different work patterns, job statuses, and perceptions of the problems, advantages, and disadvantages of the work" (Reverby, as cited in Birnbach & Lewenson, 1991, p. 111). Even as early as 1919 (Haasis, 1991), nurse leaders recognized that a good nurse not only needed hospital training but also public health nursing training. There was early recognition that the public health nursing field "wants more nurses, better equipped nurses, more clearly defined and closely coordinated work between doctors and public health nurses" (Foley, as cited in Birnbach & Lewenson, 1991, p. 133).

Today, while the majority of patients reside in the community, we deemphasize community health and public health nursing compared to acute care nursing. The emphasis needs to shift with a focus on caring for patients in the community, with some experience provided in the hospital setting.

Rights for Nurses

In the 1920s, there was hesitation on the part of many hospitals to hire nurses because they were difficult to control and were expensive (Reverby, 1987). They demanded breaks and time off. Coming from a variety of nurse training schools, they brought varying techniques, and they frequently left the job if they were not happy. Nurses often moved from job to job due to personal and professional issues, but upward mobility was difficult to achieve. In nurse training schools, excellent students were typically tracked into roles as superintendents or head nurses, while others tended to become private duty nurses (Reverby, 1987).

Then, as now, nursing was primarily a woman's occupation, while medicine was traditionally for males. Nurses were expected to sacrifice for their work and for their patients because that was the expectation of all women. In 1913, a bill was proposed to restrict the work hours of women. There was some opposition to the bill among nurses because, among other reasons, it would classify nurses as "trade workers." The California Nurses Association, which opposed the bill, stated: "Real nursing, self-sacrificing service, cannot be timed by the clock. It never has been, and it never will be" (Reverby, 1987, p. 127).

Nursing struggled to be seen as a profession instead of a trade, and to separate itself from other female occupations such as factory workers. Paradoxically, these efforts worked against the profession by excluding nursing from the public scrutiny experienced by other female workers. If nurses were viewed in the same way as female factory workers, for instance, their working conditions would have improved according to the 1913 law. As it was, wages and conditions were not reported until mid century. Nurses on the front lines of care believed that wanting an adequate wage did not conflict with the desire to provide high-quality care. The other consequence of this was that the public had little knowledge of what nursing was or should be (Reverby, 1987). There was also avoidance, in general, of any connections with women's suffrage, which further distanced the image of nursing from the rights and goals of all women.

[handwritten margin note: Trade vs. professional. # - protection vs self-sacrifice]

NOTE

We continue to encourage what I call "nurse heroics," which feeds into the image that we nurses have of ourselves as martyrs to patient care. The patient is most concerned with receiving safe and effective care. We don't seem to be able to trust each other to carry on our work while we take breaks and vacations that are necessary to our own health and well-being.

In the past, nurses were seen as members of the hospital family. As such, their work could not be regulated or assigned wages any more than could be done for a mother. The image of the student nurse as subservient was reinforced by physicians, who saw student nurses as daughters to be controlled and subordinate. Nursing students were expected to be grateful for the privilege of working in the hospital for which they received a very small stipend, not a salary. In exchange, hospitals received skilled labor that was practically free.

Later, nurse leaders recognized the need for consistency of nursing staff for the patient's benefit and for an 8-hour day to allow the nursing student time to rest and study. The nurse was expected, under the provisions of the 8-hour law, to go off duty regardless of what she was doing (Pahl, as cited in Birnbach & Lewenson, 1991). Nurses today who work in hospitals frequently work 12-hour shifts. My grandmother, who picketed in the 1920s for the move to an 8-hour day was horrified to learn that modern nurses were in favor of 12-hour days. Not only did she see this as undermining the efforts of her generation, but she could not understand how a nurse could continue to provide high-quality care for such a prolonged period.

Elitism Surfaces

In 1896, Lavinia Dock made the case for a nursing organization that avoided "the appearances of a clique" (Dock, as cited in Birnbach & Lewenson, 1991, p. 307), but advocated for a "standard of attainment, or it will be chaotic and without influence" (Dock, as cited in Birnbach & Lewenson, 1991, p. 306). When a national nursing organization was suggested, Isabel Hampton (Robb) recommended that the formation of an organization of training school superintendents precede the establishment of a national nursing organization (Reverby, 1987). From the beginning, the American Society of Superintendents of Training Schools for Nurses in the United States and Canada—later the National League of Specialty Training Schools and eventually the National League for Nursing Education (NLNE)—restricted membership (Reverby, 1987). Later, this organization created the Nurses' Associated Alumnae of the United States and Canada. This group restricted membership to schools with a minimum of 2 years of training in relatively large general hospitals. There was no intention to be all encompassing.

In 1911, the name was changed to the American Nurses Association (ANA) and membership become slightly less restrictive. Both the NLNE and the ANA intentionally included primarily middle class to upper class nurses with education from the top schools. The membership consisted mostly of self-acknowledged nurse leaders. "Working nurses" claimed that nursing superintendents should not have any control over the profession or their work and questioned how many of the superintendents had actually worked as nurses (Reverby, 1987).

Disunity Begins

This era marked the apparent beginning of disunity among nurses, which has prevented the profession from enhancing the public image of nursing and from overcoming physician paternalism. "Nursing might have been able to overcome physician hostility if it had been united itself. But the leadership's professionalizing ideology and strategy were perceived by many working nurses...as either irrelevant or in opposition to their definition of nursing and its problems" (Reverby, 1987, p. 131).

Many nurses decried the image of nursing as self-sacrificing and angelic, making the case that nursing was an honorable profession available to women and for which they could receive pay. These nurses had a distinctly different view of nursing from the nurse leaders of the day, many of whom had not worked in private practice nursing, the most common form of nursing at one time. Nurses expressed anger and resentment that they should be seen as inadequate or different because they attended small training schools or came from disadvantaged backgrounds. These nurses were initially denied the right to sit for the registration exam. Many nurses claimed that elitism separated the nurse superintendents, who saw themselves as the decision makers for the profession, from the practicing nurses. Nurse leaders were viewed as having the time and money to run organizations, while the practicing nurses had neither and could not form their own organizations.

Isabel Hampton Robb, in a speech made to the NLNE in 1897, claimed that she did not look down upon nurses from small or specialty training schools. She sought a broader education for nurses to "draw us as a profession nearer together" (as cited in Birnbach & Lewenson, 1991) because "we know that nurses are *made* not born." Hampton Robb advocated for nurses to use their intellect "so that her brain may be in good condition to understand the theory of nursing, and she may do practical work with more understanding" (as cited in Birnbach & Lewenson, 1991). Annie W. Goodrich, while speaking to the NLNE in 1912, made a plea for legislation that would define who could be called "nurse" (as cited in Birnbach & Lewenson, 1991). She asked that every nursing school be compliant with educational requirements because "the short-course school [is] a greater menace to public safety than is generally realized" (as cited in Birnbach & Lewenson, 1991).

As early as 1922, Edna L. Foley commented that nurses had reached a point where they felt that they didn't want to care for the sick but would rather teach, supervise, or inspect (1991). She made a case that "we should cease to quibble over these meaningless distinctions of title" (as cited in Birnbach & Lewenson, 1991). In 1928, Anna D. Wolf continued this dialogue, lamenting that nurses did not want to do general hospital work or bedside nursing, noting: "They feel this type of service is menial and not deserving of ambitious women....Why should our graduates feel that the very nature of general duty is undignified and not worthy of their attention, time and service?" (as cited in Birnbach & Lewenson, 1991). She stressed that nurse administrators were responsible for conveying this message by saying that the nurse is capable of more than general duty. She believed that nurse executives had to honor and value general nursing work and bedside care so that the work would be meaningful and satisfying to the nurse. She also emphasized the need for the nurse to feel that she is developing intellectually from her work and to have regular periods of rest and recreation. However, Ms. Wolf also stressed that nursing is a service and that one should willingly work overtime when necessary but receive vacation time in recompense.

This chasm between the "bedside nurse" and nurses in academic or administrative positions has continued to widen (Neal-Boylan, 2013). Partly because many nursing faculty do not maintain a clinical practice of their own, they become far removed from the day-to-day issues confronting the practicing nurse. Yet, it is largely the self-acknowledged nurse leaders—most of whom hold academic or administrative positions—who make the decisions on behalf of the profession.

Moreover, the proliferation of nursing journals and the associations that sponsor them has contributed to the disunity within the profession. As early as 1915, Sophia Palmer advocated for nursing magazines, but cautioned "against the establishment of so many of such magazines that they will not be sufficiently supported to do the most efficient work" (as cited in Birnbach & Lewenson, 1991). Her prediction has come true.

Students Are Not Well-Prepared

From the perspectives of the early leaders and the members of the nursing organizations, nursing education had to be upgraded and standardized. They believed that nurses should be considered professionals based more on their education than on their character. Long hours and hard work were seen as adversely affecting recruiting. Nurse leaders saw the necessity of improving the conditions, thus the image. In addition, there was early mention of the need to educate students to care for people of diverse backgrounds and to instill "an idea of internationalism" (Gray, as cited in Birnbach & Lewenson, 1991, p. 122). Other needs within the profession clearly resound today, such as the need for more nurses with a psychiatric mental health background and experience in emergency preparedness (Haasis, as cited in Birnbach & Lewenson, 1991). The 1918 flu epidemic helped nurses to realize the value in emergency preparedness. Today, new specialties have arisen due to fear of germ warfare and terrorist activity.

As early as 1907, nurse leaders pushed for uniformity in nursing education and a higher standard for admission (Birnbach & Lewenson, 1991). In 1930, nurse leaders were still talking about encouraging applicants of "sufficient educational background and native intelligence... They must possess those innate personal qualities which shall render them adaptable and acceptable in their profession" (Wheeler, as cited in Birnbach & Lewenson, 1991, p. 183). Claribel Wheeler went on to say, "We are admitting to our schools hundreds of young women who are personally unqualified for nursing....[We need] more careful selection of applicants" (1991, p. 183). She blamed "personality difficulties" (p. 189) for many student failures. By that she meant having an inability to accept suggestions from superiors; lacking a sense of responsibility, kindness, and sympathy; having an "overbearing attitude," (p. 189); and being unable to organize their work.

This was repeated in 1932 when D. Dean Urch emphasized that students should have "the innate capacity to learn how to solve problems, make judgments, and assume responsibilities and risks of acting on their own judgments. Certainly they should be above average in native intelligence" (Urch, as cited in Birnbach & Lewenson, 1991, p. 234). According to Urch, students should be able to withstand the physical and mental stress involved in nursing, and scientific means should be used to select students for admission. Ms. Urch decried the injustice of admitting students who were not physically and mentally fit for nursing because of the cost "in time, energy, and money" (p. 238). Frances P. Bolton felt that the typical nursing student, still a teenager, was too inexperienced in life to realistically be able to understand "the value of human life" (Bolton, as cited in Birnbach & Lewenson, 1991, p. 258).

D. Dean Urch (as cited in Birnbach & Lewenson, 1991) also discouraged keeping nursing students in school who were not suited to be nurses and encouraged linkages among schools that would avoid one school admitting a student who was dismissed from another school for inadequacy. Then as now, students frequently had no idea of what they were getting into when they applied to nursing school, but when they did enter, it was incumbent upon the faculty to encourage lifelong learning.

Even in 1900, it was recognized that students should be e[x] to the history of nursing and to business practices and law, an[d] be able to "formulate their thoughts and opinions and to expr[ess] in a business-like manner" (Walker, as cited in Birnbach & Le[wenson,] 1991, p. 206). This was reiterated in 1927 when Laura M. Gr[ant] recommended these topics as well as learning "professional, s[ocial,] civic responsibilities, nursing organizations, nursing legislation[, nursing] literature...[and] problems of supply and demand" (as cited in [Birnbach] & Lewenson, 1991, p. 226). Grant favored using case studies, [group] discussions, and individual conferences as teaching methods. L[ouise] J. Taylor argued that while trying to make nursing education le[ss hard,] educators and administrators had gone to the far extreme (as c[ited in] Birnbach & Lewenson, 1991, p. 231).

Anna D. Wolf discussed the ongoing education of staff and [the] orientation for new nurse graduates. The new nurse should be fu[lly] informed of the expectations before beginning the job and she shou[ld] be welcomed and mentored by experienced staff. She advocated for putting a great deal of time and thought into structuring orientations to aid the nurse's adjustment. Today, we still lack standardization of new nurse orientation. Many facilities don't train their preceptors or require a minimum number of hours in orientation before the new graduate is given complete responsibility for patients.

Ms. Wolf contended that if a nurse were to find that she disliked the work and could not adjust, she should be clearly told for her sake and for that of others to go elsewhere and seek other opportunities. It is doubtful that today's nursing faculty tell students they consider unsuited to the profession to leave it, and if they do, they are probably keeping that as quiet as possible! Ms. Wolf also believed that administrators should learn from the nurse's objections and use that information to improve the education of staff. Interestingly, most of the concerns nurses expressed at that time with their work continue to exist, such as "relationships between head nurses or other executive officers and staff nurses; certain undesirable combinations of work hours; certain methods of nursing procedure; rotation of service; lack of opportunity for individual expression and development" (Wolf, as cited in Birnbach & Lewenson, 1991, p. 145).

> **NOTE**
>
> *Why are we reluctant to tell an applicant or a student that he or she is not well suited for nursing? Isn't it unethical, in some respects, to encourage students who we know will be unhappy and who might actually endanger patients to become nurses? Fortunately, nurse educators are typically very careful about scrutinizing students who may be unsafe from a clinical standpoint, and most faculty I know do not hesitate to have such students repeat a course or be dismissed from the nursing program. But few acknowledge that nursing students who are in school for the wrong reasons or who do not show aptitude for nursing may also eventually endanger a patient out of lack of interest or due to inattention to detail.*

Tough Working Conditions

During the early 20th century, nurses generally did not recommend nursing to their friends and acquaintances because of the tough working conditions—"the long hours of duty, the needless repetition of much of the purely manual work, the meagerness of the theoretical work offered, and the unintelligent application of the old traditions" (Stewart, as cited in Birnbach & Lewenson, 1991, p. 165). Some recommended allowing specialization in the last year of nursing school. Nurses have always worked very hard, and up until fairly recently, they did not have the advances in technology to assist them. Even so, today's nurses still speak of hard work and arduous tasks.

Frances P. Bolton noticed that after working for some time, many nurses looked worn and tired. She supported teaching students about illness prevention and wellness for their patients and themselves, and lamented that physicians placed little emphasis on these things in favor of disease and cures. She also counseled against allowing nurses to think of themselves as martyrs because of the hard work and poor conditions. Rather, she urged that these conditions be improved to help maintain nurses' health. Interestingly, Bolton applauded the *esprit de corps* present in nursing at the time (1925), but she discouraged nurses from becoming insular, urging them to work together with others outside of nursing.

Nursing Shortage and Ancillary Staff

We find ourselves in a situation not unlike that of previous episodes in nursing history, such as in 1933, when Shirley Titus stated, "Can we doubt that change is necessary, that action is needed, when bleak and stark before us lies that grim reality, that paradoxical situation, an ever increasing army of unemployed nurses and an under nursed community?" (as cited in Birnbach & Lewenson, 1991, p. 346.) Today, there is an acknowledged shortage of registered nurses. However, it is taking longer for new graduates to get jobs than previously. Healthcare organizations want to hire less expensive, less well-trained personnel, and have resorted to once again using unlicensed staff to perform what should be done by a skilled nurse. Our communities are "under-nursed" but don't realize what they are missing by being cared for by people other than registered nurses.

With the onset of World War I, the need for nurses superseded the willingness to wait for trained, skilled nurses. Nurse leaders fought against aides who would volunteer to do nursing work. The 1918 flu epidemic further increased the need for nurses. According to nurse Isabel Stewart, this "revived again the old agitation about the 'overtraining' of nurses and the clamor for a cheap worker of the old servant-nurse type" (Reverby, 1987, p. 162). Dr. Charles Mayo of Mayo Clinic fame recommended the creation of "sub-nurses" (Reverby, 1987, p. 163), who would meet less rigid educational requirements and require shorter training than other nurses. In 1923, the Goldmark report recommended that sub-nurses be trained and licensed to care for patients with less severe or acute illnesses and work under the physician with possible supervision by the nurse.

There was opposition to this idea, although some nurses supported the concept of a worker who would answer to the nurse. Nurses were worried that the public would not be able to differentiate the untrained worker from the trained nurse (Reverby, 1987).

The profession is still dealing with this issue and has perhaps become its own worst enemy. Early in the 20th century, the call for untrained workers to supplement trained nurses arose. This was because of the insufficient numbers of trained nurses to meet the demand and because there was reluctance to pay their wages. Since then the profession has allowed programs for licensed practical nurses and nurse's aides to proliferate. We have seen the periodic use of other untrained workers to perform what should be the work of the professional nurse. We have prolonged the existence of 3 entry-level pathways into nursing: the diploma, the associate's degree, and the bachelor's degree. Confirming the fears of early nurse leaders, the public does consider almost anyone who provides care (other than a physician) to be a nurse until they are told otherwise. The nursing profession further complicated matters by eliminating a standard uniform for all registered nurses, making identification and differentiation of the professional nurse very difficult. As noted by Titus:

> We as a group must face the fact that our efforts in behalf of our profession have been diffuse rather than concentrated; we have acted individually rather than as a group, and we have dealt with our problems largely in an emotional way rather than in a rational way. (as cited in Birnbach & Lewenson, 1991, p. 347)

Conclusion

This first chapter has laid the groundwork for nursing to develop as a profession. Early nurses and nurse leaders struggled with myriad issues in their efforts to coalesce varying perspectives and interests. It will become clear as this book continues that many of the issues with which these early nurses and nurse leaders struggled remain with us today, although some may have evolved or diminished in their complexity.

PRIMARY ISSUES

Who is a nurse?

Standardizing nursing

Critical thinking

Physicians feel threatened

Lateral violence

Community health nursing

Rights for nurses

Elitism

Disunity begins

Clinical practice issues

Students not well-prepared

Tough working conditions

Nursing shortage

Ancillary personnel

References

Birnbach, N., & Lewenson, S. (Eds.). (1991). *First words: Selected addresses from the National League for Nursing 1894–1933.* New York: National League for Nursing Press.

Neal–Boylan, L. (2013). *The nurse's reality gap: Overcoming barriers between academic achievement and clinical success.* Indianapolis: Sigma Theta Tau Publishing.

Reverby, S. M. (1987). *Ordered to care: The dilemma of American nursing, 1850–1945.* Cambridge: Cambridge University Press.

Ruby, J. (1999). History of higher education: educational reform and the emergence of the nursing professorate. *Journal of Nursing Education, 38*(1), 23–27.

Chapter 2
Rising From the Depths: We Are Not Subservient (1935–1970)

My mother was 9 years old one wintry morning in 1942 and couldn't get out of bed to go to school. My grandmother, a registered nurse, anxiously examined her, fearful that infantile paralysis, later known as polio, had struck—although it did not typically do so in winter. My grandmother paid special attention to my mother's vital signs, including a high fever and the condition of her knees. There was a physician on the street where they lived who was known to make house calls. Fearing not only polio but rheumatic fever, my grandmother knew she needed to consult a physician. Dr. Bloom visited my mother and examined her gently and reassuringly. He prescribed a new drug—sulfonamide, an antibiotic that predated penicillin and was known to prevent rheumatic fever. My grandparents were poor, but an affluent friend paid the doctor and bought the medicine that ultimately saved my mother's life.

As the nascent nursing profession gained its footing, the need to carefully examine nursing education arose. War also influenced decisions about nurse preparedness. Professionalism and how nursing qualifies as a profession emerged as an important conversation. Many of the issues identified early in the century continued or evolved, and nurse leaders were challenged to develop strategies to address them.

Nurse Workload

By the 1930s, hospitals were growing in size and number, and nurses were required to supervise care that was becoming ever more complex. When hospitals took steps to group patients into units, 8-hour shifts became more possible and reasonable (Reverby, 1987). Some nurse leaders felt that shorter hours might attract more women to nursing. However, there was no definition of what a nurse's workload should be. We still argue about what constitutes a reasonable nurse workload. Those who focus attention on the matter are viewed by some as shirkers and not dedicated to the "calling" of nursing. Still, everyone complains about their workload and acknowledges that nurses often bring it on themselves.

Community Health

By 1936, according to Annie W. Goodrich, "the opportunity of the nurse in the field of health education is now generally conceded" (p. 764). Goodrich went on to say, writing for the *American Journal of Public Health*, that there was now increased focus on the educational preparation of public health nurses. She lamented the numbers of sick who could not be cared for and the births that could not be attended because of the inadequacy of funding for public health nursing. Goodrich emphasized how important prevention was to health and that all healthcare workers should be educated about prevention. She acknowledged that study of the sciences as well as liberal arts helped form the foundation for learning about preventive health and for becoming a professional nurse. Goodrich notes:

> The stultifying influences of the sometimes unpleasant procedures, repetitive almost to the point of revolt, can only be overcome by an interest and purpose that holds the attention above the drudgery of the means through which the desired end must be achieved (Goodrich, 1936, p. 768).

As in the earlier part of nursing's history, the need for a broad-based education in the liberal arts and sciences was recognized as the path toward understanding the basis behind the care nurses were providing. In addition, students from many parts of the world began coming to the United States to study (Goodrich, 1936).

In 1941, during a conference of the NLNE, the need was reiterated for public health nurses to have all the fundamental nursing education required of other nurses, with special emphasis on psychiatric nursing. In addition, it was emphasized that public health nursing should be taught by faculty with public health experience (NLNE, 1941). The Public Health Service Act was signed into law in 1944. Among other things, the law allowed for funding to train personnel specifically in public health. The law permitted nurses to be commissioned in the public health service ("Public health reports," 1944).

Although specific public health concerns and issues have changed over the years, there remains a clear place for nursing, which is still largely undervalued. While nurses serve in home and community health roles, that sort of work is often seen as "not sexy" by nursing students. I think this is because most faculty have backgrounds in the hospital and are most comfortable teaching based on their own experience. In academe, little enthusiasm and relatively little effort is put into showing students how rewarding and challenging community health work can be.

Standardizing Education

A report sponsored by the Grading Committee followed the Goldmark Report. It reported on the increasing number of trained nurses graduating from nursing schools. The report highlighted the poor quality of the education, its variability, inadequate and poorly prepared faculty and equipment, and insufficient clinical content as having a direct impact on the preparation of nurses.

The Grading Committee's work helped to decrease the number of schools and institute the requirement for a high school education prior to admission. However, there still existed much variation in schools. Many were now connected to colleges or universities, but there continued to be great variation in admission requirements and curricula.

Around this time, the Association of Collegiate Schools of Nursing was created, with the goals of working toward a collegiate level of nursing education, increasing the number of schools that were aligned with colleges and universities, and promoting new ideas in nursing education and practice. Goodrich (1936) wrote of the "dormant interest awaiting the specialists" (p. 768) who would replace the contemporary view of the nurse. By "specialist," she was referring to nurses who chose to focus on a particular area of health and medicine, just like physicians, and therefore required specialized education and training.

Emergency Preparedness

In 1940, nurses met in New York to discuss the role of nurses in the defense of the nation. The Nursing Council on National Defense was organized as a direct result of this meeting. Their first task was to explore "the nursing forces of the country in order that experience and qualifications of all nurses will be available when selecting personnel in the event of an emergency" (Haase, 1941). The council sent a survey to all registered nurses to determine nurse availability and eligibility for civilian or military service. At a conference sponsored by the National League of Nursing Education in 1941, early plans for the Red Cross Nurses Training Camp were announced and descriptions of nursing in WWI and in the Spanish American war were provided to participants. It was claimed that a lack of a national nursing organization during those wars prevented nurses from providing service at a high enough standard (NLNE, 1941).

The focus on the Red Cross shed light on the inadequacies of training presumably taking place in small hospitals and the need for nurses who worked for the Red Cross to be prepared in obstetric, medical, surgical, and pediatric nursing. It was believed that the clinical experiences provided to students in the small schools were insufficient to prepare nurses to care for the military sick or to help civilians during a disaster. It was proposed that some sort of postgraduate education be allowed to make up for the lack of adequate preparation (NLNE, 1941). Instituting refresher courses to requalify nurses to practice was also recommended.

Ancillary Staff

It was considered especially dangerous to allow standards of nursing education and practice to be lowered in part because it might pave the way for poorly trained and unsupervised "subsidiary workers" to make inroads into the profession (NLNE, 1941, p. 817). Discussion about ancillary staff, sub-nurses, or what we might today call nurse's aides or licensed practical nurses, became very intense during this period, particularly in light of impending war. The NLNE's report of the conference proceedings mention three integral elements if subsidiary workers were to be used: "careful selection, careful training and supervision, careful placement" (p. 817). Another conference speaker stressed "the need to differentiate between the functions of the professional and non-professional workers and for hospital personnel to understand this differentiation" (p. 817). There was continued discussion at the conference regarding the use of subsidiary workers—how and when they should be supervised by a nurse and which activities should be assigned to a subsidiary.

Anna D. Wolf from Johns Hopkins School of Nursing summarized the issues facing nursing at that time:

> The deleterious effect upon a good faculty who may have more than they can humanly accomplish due to the reduction of the staff, the spreading of activities so thin that good teaching is not possible; extreme difficulty in maintaining adequate and subsidiary staff to stabilize nursing care of patients in which an educational program can be carried out effectively; necessary changes in content of the curriculum; undue pressure to admit too many students for the facilities provided for learning and too many unqualified students who will later be a burden upon the community as graduate nurses; pressure to increase student nurses' hours beyond the accepted time as approved for all social groups to the extent that health may be undermined, educational program[s] may be extremely limited and a reversion to the apprenticeship method may result; financial resources diverted from educational purposes. (NLNE, 1941, p. 819)

Does this sound familiar? We continue to grapple with many of these same issues today. Among other suggestions, Ms. Wolf recommended the following potential solutions:

> There must be utilization of every means at our disposal to safeguard the standards of our schools which will produce a sufficient number of required properly qualified graduates... That we stabilize nursing service in clinical fields as far as possible through the work of auxiliary staffs including volunteer nurse's aides... That we reduce nursing to essentials and carry those essentials out to a high degree of professional efficiency....develop ways and means of caring for patients in homes through visiting nurse services... That we establish group nursing on private floors... That we give consideration to such revisions of the curriculum which may provide for a more prompt preparation of students, this to be based entirely upon high qualifications of students upon admission and in the school or upon the advance of those students who show particular aptitude in their course of study and, by virtue of that, could be graduated more promptly than others. (NLNE, 1941, p. 810)

Enhancing Rigor

Comprehensive examinations at the end of the preclinical period and at the end of each academic year, together with careful student selection and intensive orientation, were suggested methods for enhancing nursing educational rigor. The difficulty on the part of the nurse educator remains the same today: determining what really makes a good nurse—the acceptable minimum and the hoped-for maximum. Recognition was given to the need to observe how the student handles both the factors within and beyond her or his control because this ability determines the quality of the nurse's judgment. The student's "internal behavior [should be] consistent with her external behavior" (NLNE, 1941, p. 822). Katharine J. Densford from the University of Minnesota described four factors that contributed to adjustment difficulties for students (p. 822):

- Treating students as employees instead of as students

- The disparity between the ideal espoused in class and the reality of the hospital

- Inadequate opportunities for working with a variety of people

- The judgment of students based on extrinsic instead of intrinsic abilities

Students and faculty still complain about these factors. Students are often expected to know more than they do when in their clinical practica. When they don't know what the preceptor or staff expects them to know, sometimes lateral violence ensues. Conversely, students don't always attend clinical well-prepared and many do not do the necessary reading and care planning to prepare for the clinical day. Both students and new graduates speak of the differences between what they hear in the classroom and the reality of nursing practice and the lack of opportunity to engage in interdisciplinary team patient care. We often judge students on the extrinsic resources or lack thereof instead of on the internal characteristics they bring to their work. Perhaps they simply don't have the characteristics that make a good nurse! This also speaks to locus of control. Students often blame their inadequacies on outside forces and not on their own lack of commitment and preparation.

Densford also emphasized that when the student is preparing to graduate, the school has an obligation to assist in the adjustment to the working world of the nurse by refreshing the student in topics that may have been offered early in the program, issuing comprehensive examinations, and offering career guidance. She highlighted the importance of learning at the bedside and the preparation of the clinical instructor to teach students effectively.

By 1945, the profession began to consider what the profession should look like after the war. There was recognition that the coordinated efforts that gained importance during the war would also be necessary in the postwar period. In 1944, a National Nursing Committee consisting of representation from five national nursing organizations had been formed. Initial meetings focused on five major areas:

- Maintenance and development of nursing services

- A program of nursing education (professional, including basic and advanced training, and practical, or technical, nursing)

- Channels and means for distribution of nursing services

- Implementation of standards (including legislation) to protect the best interests of the public and the nurse

- Information and public relations program ("A comprehensive program," 1945, p. 707)

Interestingly, the article that discussed the planning committee and its initiatives specifically states that the program that was developed by the planning committee "relates to all nurses—professional and practical, negro and white, men and women" ("A comprehensive program," 1945, p. 707). This was a rare mention of nurses who were non-White and not female. The article, which does not list authorship, also stressed that:

> The term "practical nurse" has never been satisfactorily defined. As generally used by the public and by many doctors it means a semi-trained or self-trained person who combines nursing and household duties in the home and who performs routine nursing services in the hospital under the supervision of a professional nurse. ("A comprehensive program," 1945, p. 707)

It was acknowledged that the use of practical nurses and "other paid workers of various types" (p. 707) had been effective during the war and that they and volunteers, WACS, and Waves, should be considered alongside professional nurses when developing a comprehensive plan. The committee acknowledged "the need for study to overcome the gaps and inadequacies in prewar nursing service and nursing education which war demands have highlighted" ("A comprehensive program," 1945, p. 707). The committee recognized that some things, such as accreditation, curriculum revision, and nursing education, were national nursing issues, while others should be local or regional in scope.

Professionalism

Writing in 1945 about the professional status of nursing, Bixler and Bixler first analyzed what it meant to be a profession. As now, the differences among what were considered professions at that time were:

> In the principal objective and the body of knowledge upon which the practice rests.... The more commonly recognized professions appear to consist of those having service

> to man and society as the primary objective, though this is
> not to deny that emotional satisfactions are derived, also
> from the practice of these professions. (p. 730)

The authors argued that nursing could not boast of its own science as the medical and biological professions could and that there needed to be more emphasis on the "why" instead of on the "how" to qualify nursing as a profession. The profession needed to be both an art and a science and to utilize other sciences to fulfill this goal. They went on to say that nursing could not be a profession, by definition, without research to move it from a static state to a dynamic one and that researchers must be trained as such and not be taken for granted. Taking this a step further, the authors claimed that "those who instruct must develop a scientific attitude in students" (Bixler & Bixler, 1945, p. 732) and that therefore those who teach must also do research. Unfortunately, there are still many nurse faculty who do not engage in research and who do not instill a scientific attitude in their students.

While many university schools of nursing are working to increase the expectations of faculty with regard to scholarship, there is substantial pushback from many faculty. The typical response is that they were hired at a time when a focused program of scholarship and a required number of peer-reviewed publications were not expected, and therefore they should be more or less "grandfathered" into this new world of increased emphasis on scholarship. This argument is inadequate and harkens back to the argument used to avoid faculty clinical practice. I have also personally encountered doctorally prepared nursing faculty who no longer remember how to conduct research. When asked to advise students in thesis or dissertation work, these faculty either decline or make a mess of things. While no doctorally prepared nurse can be expected to be an expert in every research method or scientific perspective that is relevant to nursing, it is reasonable to expect that a doctorally prepared faculty be willing and motivated to refresh their knowledge to guide students effectively.

Moreover, in our effort to include evidence-based practice techniques in our nursing research courses, many faculty have relegated research methods and the rudiments of research critiquing to the back burner. Students must learn about evidence-based practice, but also understand how to critically read research even at the undergraduate level. How can they be expected to understand why we do the things we do as we diagnose and care for patients without being able to independently critically analyze the research?

Educational Preparation

Above all, Bixler and Bixler (1945) lamented that the most important factor preventing nursing from being recognized as a profession was the educational preparation that nurses received. Not only was there a great deal of variation in what constituted a nurse and what type of education was received, but what focus there was on advanced training was offered only to those who wanted to teach, supervise, specialize, or work in public health. Bixler and Bixler asked, "Is general staff nursing to be left behind in the professional evolution of nursing?" (1945, p. 732). They suggested that nurses who did desire to move into leadership positions and who were educationally prepared to do so should be encouraged in their efforts.

> The profession should definitely plan for the discovery of promising leaders and persistently cultivate their capabilities. At every turn these young women should be stimulated to develop judgment and resourcefulness and to press for responsibilities in some chosen area of nursing in line with their special interests and aptitudes. Then they should be rewarded by appointments to challenging positions. They should [begin early] to sit in the councils of the leaders and to feel themselves an integral part of the deliberations instead of being kept on the sidelines where they can participate only as spectators. Their young energies should be absorbed by having to function in complex situations in which they would have the maturing experience of making decisions and then having to take the consequences of these decisions. (Bixler & Bixler, 1945, p. 733)

Further, schools of nursing should be autonomous within colleges and universities and not be departments within other schools, for a real profession functions autonomously. Being a department rather than a school was an example of the subservience of nursing, which further prevented it from being considered a profession.

Disunity Continues

The Bixlers urged nurses to unify not only to conquer barriers to becoming a profession, but also to acknowledge that the disparate professional organizations and activities served to fragment them. This was later reiterated by Frank Lang in a 1970 article that included thoughts of various nurses and nurse leaders on the decade to come.

> Nursing, united, must react openly and concretely…or nursing will remain divisive, static, and eventually will stagnate. If this occurs, nursing will assume an inferior position in the expanding spectrum of health careers. The content and context of nursing must now relate to social sensitivity and social need, and must provide for unity among its practitioners. (Lang, 1970, as cited in Alfano et al., p. 2,122)

Finally, the Bixlers urged nurses to "adopt high ideals of freedom of action and provide opportunities for professional growth and economic security for its practitioners" (1945, p. 735).

Defining Nursing

This discussion continued into 1960, when Dorothy Nayer of Columbia University wrote of how nurses should be expert technicians but must also have "more than a nodding acquaintance with those aspects of professional nursing which embody the skills of the mind; defining, assessing, judging, and taking action on reasoned conclusions" (Nayer, 1960, p. 1,469). The article reviewed the progress made to that point by the American Nurses Association and the National League for Nursing Education, paying particular attention to a project started in 1952 by the ANA. The project sought to examine the qualifications necessary to be a professional nurse and the standards for practice.

In 1949, the interest in public health expanded into the field of geriatrics and chronic disease. Already diabetes and cancer were recognized as highly prevalent. Rheumatic fever was also among the top three diseases in several states across the country. A Commission on Chronic Illness was established. However, there were no nursing organizations associated with its establishment. Primary and tertiary prevention were emphasized, as well as the need to educate the public that chronic illness was not hopeless and that anyone with such a diagnosis was not doomed to institutionalization (Commission on Chronic Illness, 1949).

Image

Also in 1949, nurse leaders convened to discuss the pressures that were closing in on nurse educators to improve and standardize nursing education. The public believed that they had a right to dictate what nursing education should be and how the nursing shortage should be properly addressed. The American public now recognized that well-educated nurses were necessary to care for people with cancer, tuberculosis, mental health problems, and other chronic diseases. They wanted these nurses in every possible healthcare setting across the country. They also wanted nurses who could teach and nurses who could conduct research.

Nursing students questioned why some nurses could practice without formal educational preparation and pleaded for better teachers. They lamented that their teachers were burdened with their service requirements and therefore had less time to teach students. In addition, students now expected to be permitted to participate in extracurricular activities and to have social lives. It seems odd that at that time teachers were so busy doing their clinical work, they had less time to teach, while today, nurse educators complain that they are too busy with their teaching requirements to engage in any clinical practice.

Interestingly, many nurses were asking the same questions we ask today: "What are the means of recruiting nursing students?...How long should the basic professional program be? Is the present curriculum adequate? Does it meet student and community needs? How can we stimulate federal aid for nursing education?...Will clinical requirements be stated in terms of days' experience or will more adequate methods be devised to appraise student achievement and development?" (Gelinas, 1949, p. 307). Graduates were also requesting postgraduate education and continuing education opportunities that were standardized and of high quality.

At this time, physicians as well as nurses and the public expressed confusion about the varying levels of nursing preparedness. They wanted to know who was ultimately responsible for the nursing care the patient received. They sought "more competent professional nurses on whom they [could] depend to function as their representatives in their absence" (Gelinas, 1949, p. 307). Hospitals were also pressuring the profession to prepare more nurses and others (such as licensed practical nurses, aides, and clerks) to staff the hospitals. However, at the time, the hospitals were supportive of nurse educators in their efforts to better prepare professional nurses. Nursing schools that were part of colleges or universities were short of faculty due to high costs. In the effort to move away from hospital nursing schools, professional nursing education became very expensive, particularly when focused on high-quality offerings. The National Nursing Accrediting Service urged high quality and a well-rounded education.

Nursing schools faced additional challenges, chief among them the cost of providing a high-quality education. A physician who spoke at a meeting at Yale University School of Nursing recognized the courage and persistence of nurses and complained that funding for nursing education was woefully inadequate and remarkably below that which medical schools received.

> We recognize then that the doctor and the teacher are essential public servants and that the public through tax funds and private philanthropy is responsible for their adequate training.... We express our gratitude to the nursing profession by sentimental phrases and alluring posters of Joans-of-Arc with large eyes uplifted in a spirit of eager service. But only when public appreciation manifests itself in more tangible forms can nursing education and nursing service attain a position of appropriate dignity and maximum usefulness. (Winslow, 1949, p. 310)

Other healthcare professionals were providing free instruction to nursing students, and clinical instructors suffered from insufficient time and opportunity to teach students all they needed to know. There was a persistent shortage of nurse educators and nurse researchers (Gelinas, 1949).The serious shortage of nursing faculty, particularly those with doctoral preparation, continues today.

The profession continued to grow in its realization that it needed to play an integral role in educating the practical nurse and ancillary staff. At the same time, it acknowledged that a list of responsibilities of nursing roles was necessary to eliminate confusion among all the stakeholders regarding who should be or could do what. "A careful analysis of all jobs by all groups ministering to the needs of the patient will focus attention on activities which only physicians can do, on those which only graduate nurses can do, and on those which can be performed by practical nurses, hospital aides, receptionists, clerks, and others" (Gelinas, 1949, p. 310).

A Broad Foundation

Recruitment of talented, intelligent students without discrimination was an additional challenge, as was instilling in them a thirst for lifelong learning and inquisitiveness about the world beyond them. There was a concern among nurse leaders that "too many schools are turning out skilled technicians rather than competent professional nurses" (Gelinas, 1949, p. 309).They acknowledged that a broad foundation in the liberal arts was vital and that nurse educators had an obligation to continue to learn and research within and outside of nursing.

In 1953, there was further discussion regarding the role of the practical nurse and the increasing numbers of "nonprofessional nursing personnel" ("Nursing practice legislation," 1954). To protect the public, the American Nurses Association acknowledged the need for a state board of nursing and supported the trend toward mandatory licensing for all nurses. The year 1955 saw the rise of community college involvement in nursing education. The Cooperative Research Project in Junior and Community College Education for Nursing was developed under the auspices of Columbia University. The goal was to test a new type of nursing educational program whereby each college would develop its own program but would share common characteristics with the other community colleges involved in the project (Montag, 1955).

In 1958, a physician published an address he had given in *The American Journal of Surgery*. The subject of his address was the shortage of nurses and the inadequate number of professional nurses to meet demand, particularly in hospital and private duty settings. The trend at the time for nurses to go into other fields, plus the cost of education and nurses' long and irregular hours, were affecting the availability of nurses in the hospital. He countered the popular notion at the time that student nurses were being overtrained by saying:

> All of us would agree that we would prefer to have the best educated nurses possible to help us care for our patients or to care for ourselves if we were ill. The increasing complexity of medical and surgical techniques during the past decade has made the care of patients quite different and much more difficult than it was ten or twenty years ago. (Bell, 1958, p. 134)

He went on to make the argument that a practical nurse or an untrained nurse is really not as inexpensive as one would think, and that "to call a woman a nurse is not to make her such" (Bell, 1958, p. 135). He supported the need for bedside or clinical experiences for student nurses and exhorted physicians to take the time to teach student nurses and to participate in helping them gain clinical experience.

At an ANA convention in 1960, plans were made to support the future of nursing education to include "intellectual, technical, and cultural components of both a professional and liberal education" (Nayer, 1960, p. 1,471) and to promote baccalaureate education as the foundation of professional nursing. Twelve principles for nursing education were derived from theories of professional education. These were studied and reviewed, and by 1962 had been accepted broadly.

> Once nurses recognize that many changes in health needs and health care have been wrought in the past 50 years and that the society of tomorrow requires a different type of nurse than that of yesterday, they must admit that nursing education must change also. Let those who long for the "good old days" in nursing take cognizance of the many things nurses are expected to do and to understand today which were unknown in the twenties and thirties.

Let those who scoff at the need for higher education look about them and see the extent to which a college education is required, not only for most of the professions, but also for any but the most elementary jobs in the world of business. (Nayer, 1960, p. 1,471)

PRINCIPLES GOVERNING PROFESSIONAL NURSING EDUCATION

1. *The determination of standards for professional education is the responsibility of the nursing profession.*

2. *All graduates of professional educational programs in nursing shall have mastered that core of basic and applied knowledge essential for effective practice.*

3. *The requirements for curricula and methods of teaching shall be flexible in order to stimulate experimentation and to permit revision and expansion of subject matter.*

4. *Professional education should provide the student with an opportunity to develop the capacity for independent judgment in the application and advancement of nursing knowledge.*

5. *The educational program should include an opportunity for the student to expand intellectual and cultural horizons through acquiring a broad liberal education.*

6. *Responsibility for the total educational experience should rest with the faculty of the educational institution.*

7. *The standards for governing the organization, faculty, and facilities of a nursing education program should be comparable to those of other professional programs within an educational institution.*

8. *The nursing faculty should have responsibility for developing and implementing the professional education program.*

9. *Responsibility for financing professional education rests with the entire society.*

10. *Adequate and stable financial resources should be provided for the programs of professional education.*

11. *The requirements for admission to programs in nursing education should be comparable to those of other professional programs within an educational institution.*

12. *Graduation from undergraduate professional programs in nursing should qualify students for entrance to graduate programs in nursing with, generally, no further academic preparation ("Principles governing," 1962, 56–58).*

In 1965, the ANA issued its first position paper on nursing education. In issuing this paper, the ANA first declared certain assumptions (see the upcoming box). The ANA declared as its position that "minimum preparation for beginning professional nursing practice at the present time should be baccalaureate degree education in nursing" (ANA, 1965, p. 107). "Care, cure, and coordination" (ANA, 1965, p. 107) were described as the essential elements to professional nursing. In addition:

> Professional nursing practice is constant evaluation of the practice itself. It provides for an opportunity for increasing self-awareness and personal and professional fulfillment. It is asking questions and seeking answers—the research that adds to the body of theoretical knowledge. It is using this knowledge, as well as other research findings, to improve services to patients and service programs to people. It is collaborating with those in other disciplines in research, in planning, and in implementing care. Further, it is transmitting the ever-expanding body of knowledge in nursing to those within the profession and outside of it. (ANA, 1965, p. 107)

ASSUMPTIONS IN ANA'S FIRST POSITION ON EDUCATION FOR NURSING

The premises or assumptions underlying the development of the position are:

- *Nursing is a helping profession and, as such, provides services which contribute to the health and well-being of people.*

- *Nursing is of vital consequence to the individual receiving services; it fills needs which cannot be met by the person, by the family, or by other persons in the community.*

- *The demand for services of nurses will continue to increase.*

- *The professional practitioner is responsible for the nature and quality of all nursing care patients receive.*

- *The services of professional practitioners of nursing will continue to be supplemented and complemented by the services of nurse practitioners* who will be licensed.*

- *Education for those in the health professions must increase in depth and breadth as scientific knowledge expands.*

- *In addition to those licensed as nurses, the healthcare of the public, in the amount and to the extent needed and demanded, requires the services of large numbers of health occupation workers to function as assistants to nurses. These workers are presently designated nurse's aides, orderlies, assistants, attendants, etc.*

- *The professional association must concern itself with the nature of nursing practice, the means for improving nursing practice, the education necessary for such practice, and the standards for membership in the professional association.*

- *Nurse practitioner: any person prepared and authorized by law to practice nursing and, therefore deemed competent to render safe nursing care (ANA, 1965, 106–111).*

The ANA also proffered a definition of technical nursing and included the need to know when it is appropriate to act and when it is necessary to seek those who are more knowledgeable. They emphasized the need for technical nurses to be supervised by professional nurses. "It is education which is technically oriented and scientifically founded, but not primarily concerned with evolving theory" (ANA, 1965, p. 108). The ANA therefore proclaimed that the associate degree should be the minimum preparation for technical nurse and that practical nursing programs be replaced with associate degree programs for technical nurses. They went further to require that nurse's aides and orderlies receive short intensive vocational training preparation instead of on-the-job training. Many nursing traditionalists had difficulty accepting the concept of a 2-year nursing education for any nurse, but author Margaret Brown Harty saw this change as an example of innovation in nursing education (1968). The availability of adequately prepared faculty was and still is an issue regardless of the educational level at which nurses were being prepared. Harty made clear that "the two-year associate degree program in nursing is *not* the first two years of study toward a baccalaureate degree. It is a technical program in nursing, unique and complete unto itself" (Harty, 1968, p. 770).

Interestingly, the ANA acknowledged even then that we were not necessarily preparing nurses to care for patients in the appropriate settings. "More than three-fourths of the curriculums in the majority of schools continue to focus on the nursing of patients who are acutely ill and hospitalized, yet more than 90 percent of persons under health care are neither" (ANA, 1965, p. 111). Similarly, in 1968 as now, discontent and dissatisfaction of hospital staff nurses were notable and were attributed to the following:

> The traumatic impact of the gap between the real and the ideal of patient care...highly discouraging. Many of these graduates are expected to assume responsibilities for which they are not prepared. Also, they are likely to be criticized for not instituting or effecting changes in patient care practices. However, it is unrealistic to assume that four years of college education is in itself sufficient to produce a dynamic change agent prepared to assume responsibility for revision and improvement essential to the delivery of quality nursing care. (Harty, 1968, p. 770)

Graduate Education

It was at this time, around 1968, that there was increased recognition of the need for nurses to be prepared at the graduate level, both master's and doctoral. This was hampered then as it is now by insufficient numbers of nurses with foundational baccalaureate education who go on to get graduate education, thereby preparing them to be faculty to teach others who enter graduate degree programs. In addition, by this time, women had many more options for education and employment, and many of those did not require the rituals or regimentation of nursing. Targeted efforts to recruit males and people of races other than White gained momentum partly due to federal funds available for training grants for nurses. Harty recommended counseling to help prospective students avoid losing money and time by helping them to understand what they were getting into by pursuing any particular level of nursing practice education.

Despite ANA's support of replacing practical nursing with associate degree technical nursing programs, there were others—such as faculty within practical nursing programs, employers of practical nurses, and the nurses themselves—who did not agree that they required a college or university education to provide quality care. Harty declares that "the present lack of clear differentiation in the educational preparation of the graduates of the various types of programs is the Achilles' heel in the field of curriculum planning and development. As one looks to the future, one can doubt whether or not 4 years of baccalaureate education will be sufficient to prepare the professional nurse of tomorrow" (Harty, 1968, p. 772).

In 1965, a physician and a nurse educator at the University of Colorado created the first program to educate nurse practitioners (Silver, Ford, & Stearly, 1967). The first program focused on pediatrics, but programs soon developed around women's health and family health (Nuckolls, 1974). Eventually, certified nurse midwives and nurse anesthetists were also subsumed under the umbrella of advanced practice nursing. Today, clinical nurse specialists are also considered advanced practice nurses. The advanced practice roles grew out of a multiplicity of factors. These included the following:

- A manpower shortage, partly due to the Vietnam war

- A demand for primary care

- Increased access and quality (Edwards, 1974; Pickard, 1974)
- A need to better serve the underserved (Silver, Ford, & Day, 1968)
- A rise in the costs of healthcare
- The enactment of Medicare and Medicaid (Lee, 1966)
- The civil rights movement
- Increased opportunities for women (Wilson, 1994, 2003)

Back to Basics

In 1970, the *American Journal of Nursing* published the insights of several nurse leaders as they looked at the decade ahead. Their comments resonate because so much of what they discussed is still under debate today. Genrose Alfano wrote of the changing image of nursing and attributed the public's confusion regarding who was a nurse to the proliferation of aides and practical nurses. The public no longer cared about who was providing the nursing, only that it was what they required to get better. She observed:

> Some activities for which it is now not considered necessary to have a registered nurse come out [include]: to bathe, feed, toilet or position patients; to give routine medications; to take temperatures; measure blood pressures, and count pulses and respirations; to be of assistance to patients in transfer activities. One might wonder at this point if the next logical question could well be, are registered professional nurses unnecessary? (Alfano et al., 1970, p. 2,116)

Alfano called for the profession to reevaluate what patients need rather than which specific functions nurses should perform and recommended increased knowledge in the sciences, technology, and pathology. "We are so busy identifying our roles that we cannot hear the voices calling for those basic comforts that were once the very reason of our existence…We have done so well in freeing the professional nurse from activities which are 'not worthy of her skill and preparation' that she may soon find herself forever at liberty!" (Alfano et al., p. 2,116).

Minorities in Nursing

Helen Burnside and Carrie B. Lenburg encouraged open enrollment to allow students from urban areas who may be "culturally disadvantaged" (as cited in Alfano et al., 1970, p. 2,119) and to offer specialized education to those in technical nursing programs to gain knowledge in specialty areas. The latter was proposed as an antidote to the public perception that "[nurses] can be all things to all people" (as cited in Alfano et al., 1970, p. 2,119). Roy Campbell also remarked on the need to not only welcome students and nurses from minority groups, but to cease "[relegating] them to evening and night shifts where they are seldom heard or seen in the decision-making processes of nursing care" (as cited in Alfano et al., 1970, p. 2,120). Others exhorted the profession to finally bring clarity and meaning to the varying levels of nursing education.

Broadening Our Reach

Virginia Henderson foretold that nurses would become more active locally, nationally, and internationally. Consistent with her theory of self-care, she saw students as becoming more self-directed and educators more as helpers and facilitators. She supported an "expanded role" for nurses but cautioned against considering them as "physicians' assistants" (as cited in Alfano et al., 1970, p. 2,121). Ada Jacox recommended that nurses learn more about organizational structure and administration and the need for some graduate programs that specialized in developing nurse administrators.

> Although clinical knowledge is unquestionably impor-
> tant, this will not be sufficient preparation for nurses in
> the future. Nurses must become increasingly sophisticated
> about social, political, and economic factors influencing
> occupational functioning both in a specific type of orga-
> nization and more broadly, in the total society. (Jacox, as
> cited in Alfano et al., 1970, p. 2,122)

Nancy Milio encouraged renewed emphasis on community nursing and a focus on health rather than illness. She also advocated for "intergroup and interorganizational relations" (as cited in Alfano et al.,

1970, p. 2,123). This foretold our current burgeoning enthusiasm about greater interprofessional involvement. Eva M. Reese also emphasized the need to recognize that the future of nursing was in ambulatory and community settings of care with a focus on prevention. "Many, indeed most, people do not now need hospital care; for those who do, the hospital stay represents a very small portion of their total health care needs. To perpetuate a hospital-focused system, therefore, seems quite illogical" (as cited in Alfano et al., 1970, p. 2,125).

Conclusion

While nursing made significant progress toward becoming recognized as a profession, many of the concerns raised early in the century remained largely unresolved through the subsequent decades. However, it is admirable (although belated) that nurses began to recognize and correct the disparities experienced by minority nurses. Even today, however, many continue to experience discrimination in school and in the workplace.

PRIMARY ISSUES
Nurse workload
Community health
Standardizing education
Recognizing non-whites and males
What is a profession?
Educational preparation
Disunity continues
Defining nurses
A broad foundation
Graduate education
Broadening our reach
BSN required for entry into practice

References

Alfano, G., Anderson, H., Bitzer, M., Burnside, H., Lenbug, C. E., Campbell, R.,...Reese, V. E. M. (2010.) Nursing in the decade ahead. *The American Journal of Nursing, 70*(10), 2,116–2,125.

ANA. (1965). American Nurses Association's first position on education for nursing. *The American Journal of Nursing, 65*(12), 106–111.

Bell, H. G. (1958). Nursing education and the shortage of nurses. *The American Journal of Surgery, 96,* 133–136.

Bixler, G. K., & Bixler, R. W. (1945). The professional status of nursing. *The American Journal of Nursing, 45*(9), 730–735.

Commission on Chronic Illness. (1949). *American Journal of Public Health and the Nation's Health, 39*(10), 1,343–1,344.

A comprehensive program for nationwide action: In the field of nursing. (1945). *The American Journal of Nursing, 45*(9), 707–713.

Edwards, C. C. (1974). A candid look at health manpower problems. *Journal of Medical Education, 49,* 19–26.

Gelinas, A. (1949). The pressure, problems, and programs of nursing education. *The American Journal of Nursing, 49*(5), 307–310.

Goodrich, A. W. (1936). Modern trends in nursing education. *American Journal of Public Health, 26,* 764–770.

Haase, P. T. (1941, March 6). Nursing Council of National Defense: Taking National Inventory of All Registered Nurses. Rolla, ND: Turtle Mountain Star, p. 2.

Harty, M. B. (1968). Trends in nursing education. *The American Journal of Nursing, 68*(4), 767–772.

Lee, P. R. (1966). New demands for medical manpower. *JAMA, 198*(10), 165–7.

Montag, M. L. (1955). Experimental programs in nursing. *The American Journal of Nursing, 55*(10), 45–46.

National League for Nursing Education. (1941). The League considers defense. *The American Journal of Nursing, 41*(7), 816–832.

Nayer, D. D. (1960). On ANA's responsibilities. *The American Journal of Nursing, 60*(10), 1,469–1,471.

Nuckolls, K. B. (1974). Who decides what the nurse can do? *Nursing Outlook, 22*(10), 626–31.

Nursing practice legislation in 1953. (1954). *The American Journal of Nursing, 54*(9), 1,083–1,084.

Pickard, C. G., Jr. (1974). Family nurse practitioners: preliminary answers and new issues. *Annals of Internal Medicine, 80*(2), 267–8.

Principles governing professional nursing education. (1962). *The American Journal of Nursing, 62*(4), 56–58.

Public Health Reports. Public Health Service Act. (1944). *Public Health Reports, 59*(28), 468.

Reverby, S. M. (1987). *Ordered to care: The dilemma of American nursing, 1850–1945.* Cambridge: Cambridge University Press.

Silver, H. K., Ford, L. C., & Day, L. R. (1968). The pediatric nurse practitioner program. *JAMA, 204*(4), 298–302.

Silver, H. K., Ford, L. C., & Stearly, S. G. (1967). A program to increase health care for children: the pediatric nurse practitioner program. *Pediatrics, 39*(5), 756– 60.

Wilson, D. (1994, 2003). Nurse Practitioners: The Early Years (1965–1974). Retrieved from http://www.mnpa.us/NPHistory.pdf

Winslow, C. E. A. (1949). Bricks without straw. *The American Journal of Nursing, 49*(5), 310.

Chapter 3

Clinicians, Scientists, and Scholars: Separate but Equal (1970–2000)

"One must be careful with one's possessions since the cadre here seem to borrow each other's things so frequently. Strictly against training, I would think, nurse." Colonel Smith had not had to part with his treasures on our unit, I observed as I watched the very elderly patient remove the twin brushes from his metal night stand. The bristles were straight and true. The burnished golden wood fit the palm of each hand. Although a bit tremulous, he raised one brush to either side of his beautiful white hair and brushed with vigor as he no doubt had done so many times during his army career.

When he appeared satisfied with his grooming, having been assisted at bath and dress by a male aide he favored, Colonel Smith walked about 20 feet to where I stood pouring medications for Mr. Harris. Many of the men sitting in the day room of the veteran's hospital psychiatric ward observed him with curiosity as he walked, shoulders erect, arms moving rhythmically at his sides. Colonel Smith was our oldest patient. I stood quietly observing him and awaited his approach. Much to my surprise, he positioned himself alongside me to my right and extended his arm outward. "I am here to review the troops and it would be a great honor, nurse, if you would accompany me," he said.

In the 1970s, psychiatric nursing discouraged fostering a patient's delusions. But this charming aged veteran believed he was on the parade field. Was it therapeutic for him if I pretended I was there, as well? The unit I was in charge of had World War II veterans primarily. This gentleman from another era and another war (Spanish-American) had no visitors. "Colonel, I shall return the cart to the other room and join you momentarily," I said. I used this bit of time to review his chart, realizing that the troops he would be "reviewing" served our country in a war of another century. I could still recognize my patient in the sepia photograph of a young, mustachioed man wearing a soft slouch hat and leggings and soft boots, holding a very long rifle in his right hand with a water canteen at his belt. I returned to the day room and before his aide could return to prepare the 95-year-old soldier for his nap, Colonel Smith and I reviewed the troops.

The changes that occurred in healthcare in the 1960s, 1970s, and 1980s necessitated changes in nursing. More patients were surviving previously fatal illnesses and benefitting from increased access to care and advances in technology (Hobbs, 2009). Nurses needed to learn how to care for people with chronic illnesses whose life expectancies had significantly increased. Meanwhile, the nursing shortage continued to be a critical issue in the 1970s. The second Nurse Training Act was authorized in 1971, but was met with presidential opposition in later years (Wright & Widdowson, 1984).

Physicians Commit to Helping Nurses

Interestingly, the *Journal of the American Medical Association* published six objectives set forth by the American Medical Association (AMA) to demonstrate its commitment to improving the physician-nurse relationship (AMA, 1970).

- **Objective 1:** *The American Medical Association recognizes the need for and will support efforts to increase the number of nurses.* The AMA supported the "recall of inactive nurses" (p. 1,881) and affirmed its commitment to improving "the stature of nursing as a profession" (p. 1,881).

- **Objective 2:** *The AMA recognizes the need for and will facilitate the expansion of the role of the nurse in providing patient care.* The AMA acknowledged its dependence on nurses and the need to support expanded roles and responsibilities for nurses. By doing so the physician could expand his or her role to include "planner and manager of a program for comprehensive care" (p. 1,881); could "concentrate on those matters demanding his singular skill"; could allow nurses to give patients more attention so that "basic service procedures can be increased and amplified"; could allow the physician to participate in continuing education by freeing up his or her time; could provide nursing with increased recognition; and could increase the potential for home care services. Further, the nurse and physician could provide "a system of care" (p. 1,882) and increase the availability of services to the underserved. The article acknowledged that state licensure laws and practice acts allow for some skills and practices to overlap. They could be considered nursing if performed by a nurse and medicine if performed by a physician, thereby allowing for the expansion of the nursing role (as long as the nurse continued to be supervised by a physician).

- **Objective 3:** *The AMA encourages and supports all levels of nursing education.* The AMA supported directing more resources to diploma programs and enhancing associate degree programs. The AMA believed this approach had the most potential for rapid increase in manpower while encouraging baccalaureate education for those "who plan to make education or administration their life work" (p. 1,882). The AMA saw itself as taking responsibility for assisting nursing in developing the appropriate educational resources to expand its role.

- **Objective 4:** *The AMA will promote and influence the development of a hospital nursing service aimed at increased involvement in direct medical care of the patient.* In this section, the AMA noted its regret of the increased administrative responsibilities that had been placed on RNs in the hospital and acknowledged that this was negatively affecting the physician-nurse relationship. They advocated for nurse participation on medical committees instead of being "separate and distinct from hospital administration and accountable to the chief of the professional staff" (p. 1,883).

- **Objective 5:** *Delivery of medical care is, by its nature, a team operation.* While this objective as stated seems open-minded and collaborative, the explanation of the objective goes on to say that, logically, the physician—by virtue of his preparation and competence—should have "definitive legal authority in matters of medical care" (p. 1,883). However, the AMA also acknowledges that the nurse should be in charge of nursing functions and "take a logical place at the physician's side when associated with him in patient care responsibilities" (p. 1,883).

- **Objective 6:** *To implement these objectives, constructive collaboration of medicine with the various elements of the nursing profession is essential.* This objective speaks to communication with nurses via their professional organizations but also outside of professional organizations. "Efforts by the medical profession to effect a more productive relationship with nurses must embrace the total nursing community" (p. 1,883).

While these objectives could be viewed from our vantage point as still quite paternalistic and superior, they were a step in the right direction. The AMA openly encouraged its members to support the nursing profession and acknowledge the value of nurses. While the nurse-physician relationship has improved exponentially since that time, concerns about physician attitude still plague nurses in some settings. The differences are that medical education purports to encourage interprofessionalism and teamwork, and that nurses are no longer afraid of standing up for themselves or for their patients. Nurse practitioners still experience the physician's paternalistic attitude when trying to gain independent agreements to practice, and nurse anesthetists still perceive discrimination from anesthesiologists. There remain conflicts between individuals and between the professions. But as younger professionals enter the workforce from nursing and medicine, these attitudes seem to be less prevalent.

Physician-Nurse Relationship

In 1977, the National Joint Practice Commission (Institute of Medicine and National Academy of Sciences) issued three impactful statements:

- They defined collaborative practice between nurses and physicians in the hospital.

- They defined and issued guidelines regarding joint practice in primary care.

- They commented on nursing staff in the hospital.

They called for a joint practice committee equally representing nurses and physicians to establish and evaluate care. They required joint and equal representation in carrying out administrative duties, providing continuing education, and meeting standards. Mutual acceptance and respect for each other's judgment was to be expected. "Each professional brings a different approach and additional information and expertise to the setting that the other professional recognizes, values, and is unable to provide alone" (National Joint Practice Commission, 1977, p. 21). The message, while enforcing the necessity of collaboration and respect, still maintained that there are key differences between nurses and physicians:

> Although both nurses and physicians concern themselves with diagnosis, treatment, disease prevention, and the maintenance of health, physicians tend to bring a diagnostic and therapeutic perspective to the medical needs of patients, while nurses tend increasingly to bring health-oriented and educational perspectives to the physical, emotional, and social needs of patients. (p. 21)

Research and Policy

The 1970s brought increased interest in and emphasis on nursing research and grant acquisition. Research turned from studies focused on qualifications for practice in the 1950s and 1960s to the specifics that define quality such as cost, accessibility, and outcomes. "Matters of research interest include the effects of nursing practice on early discharge, lack of complications, early return to work, incidence of hospital readmissions, health maintenance, and prevention of illness" (Gortner, 1973, p. 1,052). Interest in interdisciplinary studies and sophisticated research methods had grown by this time. Specialty grants were offered in the late 1950s through the mid 1960s that allowed faculty in schools with graduate programs to acquire the resources needed to conduct quality research and achieve doctorates. Gortner exhorted nurses to direct research efforts toward teaching and learning practices and historical research, and to expand research about nursing practice beyond descriptive and exploratory studies.

By 1989, nursing research had "become an accepted and respected pursuit in universities and colleges that prepare nurses to degree and diploma levels" (Chibuye, 1989, p. 326). However, it remained largely focused on topics related to acute care. Chibuye contended that nursing research was "often irrelevant to the needs of the greater population" (p. 326). She lamented that little research was being done at the primary care level, particularly with regard to access, nutrition, sanitation, and education. She blamed nurse leaders for remaining hospital oriented, nursing education for stagnating, and "nurses [for] not having taken deliberate steps to ensure that all nurses at all levels acquire the necessary knowledge and skills in primary healthcare, including assisting them to adopt appropriate attitudes" (p. 327). She wrote that nurses, in their eagerness to be considered professional and more like those in the medical profession, had become more rigid, with the result of nurses caring more about their image than about the patients. She claimed that to affect health policy, nursing education, practice, and research had to change.

> The two vital questions are "Where do we go from here?" and "How do we influence the work of nurses?" In my opinion, the various nurses' groups do not collaborate enough, thus creating too few opportunities to learn from each other (p. 328). The challenge nurses must meet is to ensure that our practice is recognized by bureaucrats and that our knowledge reaches the right people. (p. 329)

Nancy Milio (1989) expanded on this theme by describing the types of timely policy questions that nursing needed to address. She stated that with regard to policy, nursing had been focused on professional issues, but that nursing needed to move beyond nursing issues to address broader policy. Doing so would require changes in how nurses think and prioritize. She recognized the importance of discussing policy in the classroom and in devising clinical placements that were policy oriented.

The Task Force on Cost, Quality, and Access (TFCQA) was endorsed by the ANA in 1989 with the charge of devising a response to the healthcare crisis and a direction for the ANA. The Task Force identified the following areas of concern: access, cost, quality, and the healthcare delivery system. In 1991, ANA issued a statement and a proposal for changes in public policy. *Nursing's Agenda for Healthcare Reform* called for a change in the delivery of care that would be more community-based, patient-focused, and with emphasis on caring and consumer accessibility. This was widely endorsed by nursing organizations and led to policy statements that further elaborated nursing's position (Trotter Betts, 1996).

The 1990s saw a significant increase in the profession's involvement in politics and policy. Cohen, Mason, Kovner, Leavitt, Pulcini, & Sochalski (1996) described the stages it had taken to get the profession to that point and the work that would be necessary to continue on that trajectory. By 2000, the International Council of Nurses (ICN) had initiated various projects to involve nurses in policymaking throughout the world. The recognition that nurses the world over had many of the same issues prompted projects in leadership and policy development. The ICN was working hard to achieve better healthcare around the world.

Given our current dedication to and advances in global healthcare, it becomes even more necessary to educate nurses to be well-rounded men and women of the world. Emphasizing the importance of reading broadly, being aware of what's going on in the world, and understanding topics outside of nursing can only help better prepare nurses for the world stage. It is important that students write and speak well and present themselves in a professional manner so they will be viewed as professionals and leaders by our colleagues across the globe.

Care Delivery

The 1970s reintroduced the concept of primary nursing. The model placed an assignment of patients under the care of one nurse, who ensured that all the patient's needs were met. Many nurses had become disillusioned with functional and team nursing and supported the notion that primary care nursing would reduce fragmentation and ensure individualized care. It was viewed as a solution to short staffing and nurse burnout. Manthey et al. (1970) "found that the team nursing approach, when applied to the day-to-day work of a nursing unit, required so many compromises in basic theory that it was rendered virtually nonfunctional (p. 68)…The philosophy of primary nursing is grounded on the staff nurse's acceptance of personal responsibility—on responsibility not being shared" (p. 77). The authors therefore challenged nurse faculty to:

> Educate each student in the area of personal awareness and the way she relates to others as well as in the comprehension of facts or material relevant to nursing, and to help her to develop the ability to make valid judgments, to determine priorities, and to act on her decisions with some degree of assurance. (p. 80)

Nurses had been doing primary nursing since well before they knew what primary nursing was. The nurse was responsible for one or more patients and every aspect of their care. Team nursing had spread this responsibility among nurses. It is interesting that the profession saw the need during this period to name their original patient care model and to ascribe all sorts of attributes to it over team nursing. Since this time, nursing has tried several types of models with none being deemed ideal. Further, despite the contention that 12-hour shifts would ensure consistency of care, patients still encounter many different nurses during any one brief hospital stay. As a profession, we often identify what will work effectively in theory, but fail to implement it in a way that will benefit us or our patients.

Minorities in Nursing

The public stereotype of a nurse remained the traditional nurse—caring, but typically not very intelligent or capable of being autonomous (Fry, 1983). In the early 1970s, however, men began to have more of a presence in nursing. Prior to Nightingale, men had served in nursing roles, but the advent of Victorian sensibilities defined nursing as natural to women and paternalism as natural to male physicians. In addition, pay was relatively poor, and men could obtain higher-paying jobs—at least until the Great Depression, when the draw of a free education attracted some men to the profession. In 1971, the American Assembly for Men in Nursing was formed to combat discrimination against men and to recruit and support male nurses (Evans, 2004). The military, however, was more progressive, and included a significant number of male nurses in the Army Nurse Corps (Evans, 2004). For a long time, while male nurses assumed leadership positions, they were banned from obstetric practice. Concerns centered around the potential for molestation, the need for chaperones, and the likelihood that female patients would object. Men were traditionally more welcome in psychiatric clinical environments (Evans, 2004).

Men still frequently encounter discrimination in nursing and often find themselves being called "doctor" by patients who automatically assume that because they are male, they must be the doctor and not the nurse. I think that most nurses would agree, however, that the addition of men in nursing has enhanced the profession. Men as a group seem to have less patience with many of the annoying trivialities with which nursing has struggled and seem more likely to question things we've always done a particular way. They expect respect and are not willing to assume a posture of the traditional subservience with which many female nurses seem to be ingrained.

The 1970s was also a time of increased awareness of the sub-rosa discrimination against minorities, particularly Black people, in nursing (Miller, 1972). A small study (Winder, 1971) in 1971 had concluded that Black girls did not choose nursing because they had no Black role models. Michael H. Miller questioned this conclusion, which was based on 32 high school students: "Such a lie of thinking presupposes that Blacks have some decisive cultural end distinct from, or even opposed to, that of whites" (p. 249). Miller contended that regardless of race, people share many of the same values and seek the same goal: "material possessions" (p. 25). He conducted his own study of 331 beginning nursing students in associate degree programs in the Mid-South. The students were in the first week of orientation and had no previous nursing education. Of the 331 students, 112 were Black and 219 were White.

He found that although Black students chose the school they attended primarily based on perceived quality or convenience, White students valued convenience over other factors. Black students chose to enter nursing directly after high school, while White students delayed entering. Consequently, the White students tended to be older and to have had more experience in a medical setting as a nurse's aide or volunteer. Interestingly, more of the Black students were male than among the White students.

Not surprisingly, family income was higher among Whites. Most of the students paid for their own education. However, despite a lower income among Black students, the White students were more likely to have full scholarships, while Black students had either partial scholarships or loans. This among other things appeared to be based on discrimination against Blacks.

Notably, with just four exceptions, there were no statistically significant differences between groups of students regarding the following variables:

- Decision to become a nurse
- Relationship of nursing to other professions,
- Knowledge of and perception about the nature of the nursing profession
- Future career orientation (Miller, 1972, p. 255)

Both groups viewed the profession as prestigious, focused on helping others, and possessing some authority and responsibility. Interestingly, the majority of participants wanted to work in a hospital full time and expected to continue their education beyond the associate's degree (Miller, 1972, p. 257). Overall, Miller contended that his data demonstrated that there was very little difference in attitudes regarding nursing between the groups. He recommended changing recruitment strategies and dispelling the notion "that Blacks value professional nursing less than whites, and thus Blacks are to blame for their underrepresentation" (p. 262).

Racism continued to be an issue in the 1990s. As Barbee (1993) stated:

> Today the racial bias in nursing is demonstrated in the small numbers of black registered nurses and black nursing students and the almost total absence of black nurses' contributions in nursing texts. As a result, black nurses are marginalized in the "caring" profession. (p. 346)

She went on to say that it wasn't only Black nurses who were the subjects of racism, but Latina, Asian, and Native-American nurses as well. "Because nursing is based on concepts of empathy and labor, nurses believe that they see all people the same" (p. 349).

Nursing educators, nursing organizations, and granting bodies are making a concerted effort to increase diversity within nursing programs and in the nursing workforce. We have a long way to go, however. As we expand our efforts, it is incumbent upon us to help students recognize and appreciate all diversity. We are all diverse, depending on one's perspective! While necessary, the conversation about diversity in recent years may increase the risk of some people thinking that there are "others," rather than appreciating that each person brings a fresh perspective by virtue of his or her own unique experiences.

The Nursing Shortage

The nursing shortage attained crisis proportions in the 1970s. Just as today, there were plenty of nurses, but there were many gaps in services that nurses were not filling (Kalisch & Kalisch, 1980, p. 141).

> Finding qualified nurses is no longer the problem only of poor or isolated regions, but has become the headache and worry of nursing administrators, hospital administrators, and physicians all over the country. Nurse recruitment has become a permanent administrative problem for hospitals and nursing homes, and professional nurse recruiters have been hired to ease the problem.

Nurses were complaining about the working conditions of the hospital related to insufficient staffing. Kalisch & Kalisch noted, "If nurses want to advance in their profession and to earn more money, they must quit patient care in favor of administration or teaching." They continued: "Even more nurses quit when they can no longer tolerate working 12- and 16-hour shifts and knowing their patients are not receiving good care" (p. 142). Nurses complained then, as they do now, that there was no time to provide emotional support or teach patients (Kalisch & Kalisch, 1980). Despite this, the Carter administration, including the Department of

Health and Human Services, favored reducing federal funding for nursing education. A lack of understanding, possibly based on misinformation, was credited for the administration's skewed perspective regarding the supply and demand for nurses (Kalisch & Kalisch, 1980).

In the 1980s, the need to control rising healthcare costs drove the direction of nursing. Roxanne Spitzer (1983) wrote that if nurses were to be proactive about cost containment, they must justify the work they do and develop alternatives such as flexible scheduling and increased use of the licensed vocational or practical nurse.

The nursing shortage in the 1980s was a reflection not only of cost containment but also of hospital working conditions, the increased variety of professional options open to women, the prospective payment system, and opposition by organized medicine to nursing's efforts to expand its purview (Iglehart, 1987). While the AMA may have once supported the expansion of nursing roles (as discussed in Chapter 2, "Rising from the Depths: We Are Not Subservient [1935–1970]"), they felt increasingly threatened—in particular by advanced practice nursing roles. Even today, many continue to question APRN autonomy while conducting highly satisfying one-on-one relationships with the APRNs with whom they work.

Despite earlier recommendations to cut funding to nursing education, the Presidential Commission on the Human Immunodeficiency Virus Epidemic warned that the nursing shortage might jeopardize the care of people with AIDS. As a result, the commission recommended increasing federal funding for student loans, employer support, and incentives to encourage nurses to pursue baccalaureate and master's degrees and other similar measures (Brennan, 1988).

Linda Aiken (1981) recognized that hospital nurses were dissatisfied and attributed this to the following:

- The "transfer of technology from physicians to nurses" (Aiken, 1981, p. 325) without a change in nurse authority

- The decreased accessibility of physicians due to lifestyle changes

- The increase in patient acuity in the hospital without "recognition of the importance of the nurse's role in the new level of clinical decision making required by these very sick patients" (p. 325)

- The multiplicity of physician specialists, requiring nurses to comply with orders from several stakeholders, and the resulting fragmentation of care

- Increased responsibility for the coordination of patient care without concomitant authority to deploy or redirect support services (p. 325)

- Changes in career aspirations for nurses who now wanted to invest time and energy in full-time career trajectories and who no longer saw the hospital environment as a short-term necessary evil

These factors, combined with the nursing shortage and improvements in nursing education, influenced the public's expectations of the profession. Aiken saw the relationship among nurses, hospital administrators, and physicians, and the redefinition of nursing roles, as key to solving these problems.

Dr. Margretta Styles, President of ANA (ANA, 1988), commented that the nursing shortage prompted numerous attempts at quick fixes but also resulted in a long-overdue meeting of the major national nursing organizations. She proposed five priorities for the profession:

- "Sharpen[ing] and maintain[ing] our sense of direction" (p. 551)

- "Strengthen[ing] the ANA and its constituent members and our leadership within all of organized nursing" (p. 551)

- Improving working conditions

- Protecting and enlarging the scope of practice

- Striving to unite nurses throughout the profession

She predicted that the specialty groups in nursing would join together to form powerful coalitions (Styles, 1990).

There doesn't seem to be a unified, clear sense of direction for the profession, probably due to the fragmentation of nursing organizations and their priorities. Dr. Styles's five priorities have not come to fruition, and rarely have specialty groups joined together to form coalitions. It is fascinating that more than 25 years later, we have been only marginally successful in accomplishing any of them.

Redefining Nursing

Changes in healthcare, increasing healthcare costs, and budget cuts forced nursing to redefine itself. Nurses had to prove their value in dollars. While changes in the economy in the 1980s were largely viewed as negatively affecting healthcare, nurses were given the opportunity to participate more fully in healthcare policy and to influence how to provide quality care at a lower cost (Wright & Widdowson, 1984).

To a stormy reception, the ANA defined nursing in its first iteration of the *Social Policy Statement* (SPS) in 1980. The emphasis on treating conditions rather than diseases angered many, particularly nurse practitioners who were struggling to promote their identity and value (Hobbs, 2009). Defining nursing for the public had become difficult in light of the rapidity of change and the variety of skills. Once again, a relatively small group of nurses spoke for the entirety of the profession; the result was a loss of ANA members and a threat to the viability of the organization.

Elitism and Disunity Continue

This elitism resurfaces repeatedly throughout nursing's history. One could argue that any nurse can choose to become an active member of a professional organization and thereby influence decisions that will affect the profession. In theory this is true. However, in practice, it is unrealistic to expect many nurses to pay the exorbitant membership fees required by many organizations. In addition, while efforts have been made for some organizations to work together toward a common goal, these efforts are typically temporary and sporadic. The 3,000,000 nurses in the United States do not belong to one organization, but to none or several, thereby fragmenting any substantive political or policy-making power we might have.

Moreover, how many of the small number of nurses who are making the decisions for the profession are engaged in current clinical practice, and how long has it been since they were responsible for a patient? Can they competently speak to the issues confronted by the bedside nurse—

here defined as a nurse who engages in any kind of direct patient care on a regular basis?

In the 1970s and 1980s, the increasing number of nurse specialty organizations competed with the ANA for members (Hobbs, 2009), resulting in the splintering of nursing influence and image. Rather than becoming fewer and more united since that time, there continue to be many nursing organizations that often work at cross purposes.

The ANA task force charged with developing the definition of nursing in 1980 decided that the term "nurse practitioner" should refer to all professional nurses (Hobbs, 2009, p. 10). This caused consternation and confusion among nurse practitioners who were working hard to obtain recognition as advanced practice nurses. In the latter half of 1980, the ANA task force attempted to revise the SPS based on the comments it had received from nurse constituents. The changes clarified that nurses without advanced education could specialize, but that a specialist possessed advanced education. In other words, a nurse could choose to enter a specialty area of nursing without obtaining certification, but could not consider himself or herself a specialist. ANA certification was considered necessary for all levels of specialization. There was no change in the definition regarding the treatment of disease. The ANA stood firm that this was not a nursing role. In 1981, the approved definition stated that "nursing is the diagnosis and treatment of human responses to actual or potential health problems."

Shortly after the release of the definition, the ANA rescinded this portion of the definition. According to Hobbs (2009), the change came too late, because by then, nurse practitioner organizations had emerged and defined nursing practice for themselves. In 1982, the ANA solicited well-known nurse academics for their support and assistance in disseminating the statement. Once again, nurses who were not actually engaging in nursing practice—and perhaps had not for some time—were attempting to represent practicing nurses (Hobbs, 2009).

> Many of the nurses involved in the creation of the SPS were removed from practice, and the exclusion of practicing nurses meant that the information practice itself did not reflect the current priorities of nurses' work. Their

attempt was largely unsuccessful because they ignored the needs of those who delivered nursing care and would ultimately decide the success of the SPS. (Hobbs, 2009, p. 15)

The Baccalaureate Degree

The continued fragmentation of nursing education in the 1980s served only to undervalue the baccalaureate degree despite attempts by the ANA to make it the minimum requirement for entrance into the profession (Igelhart, 1987). While the ANA had called for the baccalaureate to be the professional degree as far back as 1965, this goal had still not been achieved. Once again, the profession has mandated the BSN for professional nurses. The Institute of Medicine's Future of Nursing report (2010) supports this and recommends that nurses work to the fullest extent of their education.

Graduate Education

Changes in healthcare heralded the need to acquire advanced skills and knowledge. Practice doctorates in nursing began to take shape in the late 1970s, when Case Western Reserve University opened the first program on the heels of the emergence of nurse practitioner programs (Hathaway, Jacob, Stegbauer, Thompson, & Graff, 2006). It wasn't until much later that the American Association of Colleges of Nursing (AACN) took steps to closely examine this new phenomenon.

The 1990s also brought increased recognition of nurse practitioners and clinical nurse specialists. NPs and CNSs could bill Medicare for their services, but in collaboration with physicians. They could bill only for the types of services a physician would provide, not for preventive or wellness services, and payment would be at 85% of the physician rate.

Conclusion

By the new millennium, nursing had collectively accomplished many great things. Significant strides had been made in medicine and healthcare. People were living longer and required different models of care. Physician organizations had begun to recognize the need for and value of professional nurses.

Nurses had become engaged in research and policy and were influencing the delivery and shape of healthcare services. The nurse practitioner role had gained momentum and forever changed the view of nurses from handmaidens to autonomous expert clinicians. Yet, fundamental problems continued to plague the profession, including a shortage, elitism, and fragmentation of nursing education and organizations.

PRIMARY ISSUES

Increasing survival rate

Chronic illnesses

Physicians commit to helping nurses

Research and policy initiatives take shape

Changing care delivery models

Men and minorities in nursing

Nursing shortage

Redefining nursing

Elitism and disunity continue

Continued fragmentation of nursing education

Development and recognition of nurse practitioner programs

BSN required for entry into practice

References

Aiken, L. H. (1981). Nursing priorities for the 1980s: Hospitals and nursing homes. *American Journal of Nursing, 81*(2), 324–330.

American Medical Association. (1970). Medicine and nursing in the1970s: a position statement. *JAMA, 213*(11), 1,881–1,883.

American Nurses Association. (1988). ANA delegates "march" on crucial issues. *AORN Journal, 48*(3), 551–558.

Barbee, E. L. (1993). Racism in nursing. *Medical Anthropology Quarterly, 7*(40), 346–362.

Brennan, L. (1988). The battle against AIDS: A report from the nursing front. *Nursing, 18*(4), 60–64.

Chibuye, P. S. (1989). Nursing in action: Nurses' influence in research and health policy development. *Journal of Professional Nursing, 5*(6), 326–329.

Cohen, S. S., Mason, D. J., Kovner, C., Leavitt, J. K., Pulcini, J., & Sochalski, J. (1996). Stages of nursing's political development: Where we've been and where we ought to go. *Nursing Outlook, 44,* 259–266.

Evans, J. (2004). Men nurses: A historical and feminist perspective. *Journal of Advanced Nursing, 47*(3), 321–328.

Fry, S. (1983). The social responsibilities of nursing. *Nursing Economics, 1*(1), 61.

Gortner, S. R. (1973). Research in nursing: The federal interest and grant program. *The American Journal of Nursing, 73*(6), 1,052–1,055.

Hathaway, D., Jacob, S., Stegbauer, C., Thompson, C., & Graff, C. (2006). The practice doctorate: Perspectives of early adopters. *Journal of Nursing Education, 45*(12), 487–496.

Hobbs, J. L. (2009). Defining nursing practice: The ANA policy statement, 1980–1983. *Advances in Nursing Science, 32*(1), 3–18.

Iglehart, J. K. (1987). Health policy report: Problems facing the nursing profession. *New England Journal of Medicine, 317,* 646–651.

Institute of Medicine. (2010). *The future of nursing: Leading change, advancing health.* Washington, DC: National Academies Press.

Kalisch, P. A., & Kalisch, B. J. (1980). The nurse shortage, the president, and the congress. *Nursing Forum, XIX*(2), 138–164.

Manthey, M., Ciske, K., Robertson, P., & Harris, I. (1970). Primary nursing: A return to the concept of "my nurse" and "my patient." *Nursing Forum, IX*(1), 65–84.

Milio, N. (1989). Developing nursing leadership in health policy. *Journal of Professional Nursing, 5*(6), 315–321.

Miller, M. H. (1972). On Blacks entering nursing. *Nursing Forum, XI*(3), 248–263.

National Joint Practice Commission. (1977). Three statements from the National Joint Practice Commission. *Supervisor Nurse, 8*(11), 20–21.

Spitzer, R. B. (1983). Legislation & new regulations. *Nursing Management, 14*(2), 13–21.

Styles, M. (1990). Eyes on the future: Will the profession unite? *The American Journal of Nursing, 90*(10), 83.

Trotter Betts, V. (1996). Nursing's agenda for health care reform: Policy, politics, and power through professional leadership. *Nursing Administration Quarterly, 20*(3), 1–8.

Winder, A. E. (1971). Why young Black women don't enter nursing. *Nursing Forum, 10*(1), 57–63.

Wright, J., & Widdowson, R. (1984). The effect of new federalism on nursing. *Nursing Forum, XXI*(1), 9–11.

Chapter 4
What Are We Doing Right?

It's hard to recall how I traveled to work. Probably by bus, as the age of street cars had passed by 1954. I was rather getting a kick out of working at the hospital that had figured so colorfully in my childhood. It was there that my mother had been in charge of the emergency room. I worked in the "clinic," which, at that time, indicated the area in which we saw indigent patients. It was the beginning of the migration of Latinos, particularly Cubans, to New York.

A beautiful, very young Mrs. Guzman was my next patient in obstetrics. She spoke no English, and a tender young man with barely a moustache on his worried face translated during her appointment. The physician who came into the room, Dr. George Papiniculau, really embodied the term "Greek god." He was quite tall and handsome, perhaps in his early sixties. He was at this inconsequential Brooklyn hospital visiting or perhaps lecturing. In any case, Dr. Papiniculau treated Mrs. Guzman with the same courtesy as I assumed he would the crown heads of Europe. I assisted him with a Pap smear and was enthralled.

During this same period at the clinic, I would join other nurses for lunch in the staff dining room. Meals were served and everyone was seated in a very hierarchical way. The physicians had their own area, so designated by signage; the nursing "aristocracy" had theirs; and the staff had their own for a 30- to 45-minute break. However, one elderly gentleman defied the classification and sat with the staff nurses, talking merrily in accented Hungarian English. He watched a nurse knitting and wanted instruction. He was a curmudgeon Jewish grandpa who also happened to be the renowned pediatrician Dr. Bela Schick. I never forgot the affection he demonstrated to the nurses. At this time, the hospital also acquired the presumed world authority on clinical medicine, Dr. Isidore Snapper. He would be chief of medicine and so highly regarded that a new building was designed and subsequently named for the great clinician. My mother was especially impressed by his appointment. Here was another prominent Jewish physician who had survived the holocaust.

According to the survey responses (see this book's introduction), there are many things we are doing well with regard to education, practice, and policy. However, as will be clear in the next chapter, there is still much room to improve in all of these areas. This chapter, along with Chapter 5, "What Are We Doing Wrong?" and Chapter 6, "Nurses Propose Solutions to Education, Practice, and Policy Issues," will be divided into three sections: "Education," "Practice," and "Policy." Nonetheless, it is important to recognize that there is a great deal of overlap between and among them.

Education

There have been a lot of changes in nursing education during recent years. Nurses who responded to the survey had a lot to say about what they liked and didn't like about how we are educating new and graduate nurses. This chapter presents their thoughts on what we are doing right.

Multiple Pathways and Program Variety

A surprising number of nurse respondents applauded the multiple options for entry into the profession. "Nursing Education is constantly changing to accommodate the changing health environment," said one respondent. They liked that working nurses can move through the educational system to obtain advanced degrees. One respondent noted, "Even though we get criticized for having multiple entry points into the practice, this may be the only way women with families are able to be educated."

Our efforts to enable seamless progression are recognized and appreciated. There is "easier entry from 2- to 4-year programs." Among the myriad educational options are many that are online. These offer flexibility. "There are college programs available and accessible at all levels," observed one respondent. Schools have clearly made inroads in both the flexibility and affordability of nursing education. As one respondent wrote, the profession "helps mature students to navigate school." However, several other nurses complained about the high cost of education. (This is discussed further in Chapter 5.) Another added:

> Nursing is beginning to have an impact on the idea that the BSN should be the first entry point into nursing...Master's entry-level programs as a starting point to becoming an RN is a brilliant move into raising the perception that nursing is a professional career, not an hourly occupation.

Excellent Education

Many nurses are pleased that the profession is requiring the BSN and hope that this time, we really mean it. Nurses value the education they receive and appreciate the high standards and high expectations set by faculty. One praised the "focus on nursing assessment," while others wrote of the "high expectations in performance," particularly in BSN programs, and the "high standards of excellence." Others wrote positively of the "strict accreditation requirements" and the need to "keep up [with] current standards of practice." They are happy that the profession "sets high standards for accrediting colleges to teach nursing."

As will be discussed in Chapter 5, many more nurses are concerned that our programs are not rigorous enough. Despite a few nurses who praised the "high standards of dress and competence," many nurses feel that "students and nurses look and act unprofessionally."

Nurses wrote of specific courses they feel have prepared them well to function effectively, such as the following:

- "General pathophysiology"
- "Education on body systems and how they work together"
- "Lots of anatomy and physiology classes"
- "Psychology of chronic diseases"
- The "psychosocial aspects of care"

Others were glad they learned about pharmacotherapeutics, medication management, and had a background in the liberal arts. Interestingly, some nurses wrote of learning about "diversity in patient care," "acculturation," and "patient sensitivity."

Many nurse respondents were happy about the "constant reminder of EBP [evidence based practice]" and having learned about "nursing research." Scholarship and research appear to be important components of nursing education, and were mentioned many times in addition to patient-centered care, care of the family, and the focus on patient teaching.

Many nurses feel that, in general, schools prepare students well for the state board exam and are pleased that many opportunities exist to obtain certification. The profession "encourage(s) national certification" and "encourages certification in specialty areas." One nurse said:

> They are trying hard to carve out a space for nursing to be accepted as a professional practice instead of an hourly technical occupation. A good comparison is an engineer versus a technician, or a software engineer versus a computer programmer. Although I think nursing is still struggling to create this important distinction.

Specialization and New Programs

Nurses are pleased that there is a variety of options for specializing in nursing. Said one nurse, "[I like the] options to specialize: administration, clinical specialist, educator." Nurses can choose to work in any number of settings and can specialize in particular clinical areas. One nurse observed that some schools are now "providing information on the variety of health settings available, not just hospital nursing." There are also "new programs focusing specifically on [the] care of veterans," for example.

Improvements in Clinical Experiences

Several nurses acknowledged the efforts of nurse educators to recognize and improve student clinical experiences. They have benefited from "strict student-to-faculty ratios in the clinical setting," "increasing focus on mentorship," "availability of people to answer questions [and] concerns," and "a wide variety of preceptorships [and] observational rotations to give students insight to various areas." Students appreciate when "instructors who are working as an instructor and regular floor nurse [have] current expertise" and when "practicing nurses [are] used for precepting students."

Some have experienced a "variety of clinical settings, procedures learned with observation skills or classmates reports, regarding nurse responsibility, [and] patient education," and have been able to "get an opportunity to try many areas of nursing." As will be clear in Chapter 5, however, many more nurse respondents believe we have a long way to go to improve student clinical experiences.

Dedication of Nurse Educators

Some nurses recognized that "nursing professors are very dedicated and passionate in teaching. Otherwise they [can] make more money working as a staff RN." They also recognized that "professors are wonderful and strongly supportive of students." Another nurse said:

> For the most part, I believe we attempt to instill the "true meaning of nursing" in our students. We do this by continuing to respond to patients holistically. And to do that we as faculty respond holistically to our students.

Innovation

Several nurse respondents praised the profession's efforts to keep up with changes in healthcare and to welcome innovation and creativity in nursing education. One respondent noted, "We try to stay creative in how we approach educating future nurses while simultaneously responding to the current demands of the profession." The profession appears to be "listening" to employers and is attempting to give them what they need. Several nurses cited the increased emphasis on nursing informatics as an example of innovation in education.

Several nurses wrote in praise of the "incorporat[ion] [of] new technologies, such as 'smart' manikins," the drive to "integrat[e] technology into education," and simulation labs and simulation training. "We are using simulations more to enrich the students' knowledge base and comfort with skills."

Practice

Survey respondents found a lot to praise about current nursing practice. There is increasing awareness of "job opportunities...[and] no longer [being] stuck either working in hospital settings or [the] school system." One respondent noted, "A nurse can work in a variety of locations other than the traditional hospital setting." There are "business opportunities [in] nurse-driven clinics [and] hospices." Many expressed appreciation for the "RN residency programs available for new graduates" and "residency orientations."

Continuing Education

The profession encourages continuing education, as well as staff and patient education. It also "encourages nurses to advance in level of practice via certifications or degrees." We "nurture a passion for the profession of nursing." There are many opportunities to obtain continuing education units and "RN refresher classes, for those out of practice for family [or] health reasons." Another praised the "ongoing nursing education so that professionals can continue to learn and fostering the idea of continuous learning throughout our careers." Many nurse respondents listed the emphases on lifelong learning, continuing education, returning to school, and obtaining advanced degrees as things the profession does well.

Provide Quality Care

Some nurses commented on the "flexibility with no retirement age for nurses" and that the profession "continually works to develop working conditions that are attractive and optimal for RNs." Nursing "drives much of [the] health and wellness focus" and "encourages community involvement."

Nurses report that "home healthcare has improved in the past few years," "nursing practice is everywhere in society," and there is more emphasis on care planning, caregiver needs, "caring about patients," and "communication with families." Nurses "car[e] for people in crisis," "car[e] for the whole patient," and "instill commitment, morality, human compassion, values, and caring." We "truly car[e] for patients and put them first," said one respondent. Nurses "provide good bedside care if time allows" and "provide safe care" that is of high quality. We "comfort patients [in] pain."

Several nurses wrote of our commitment to quality. We "strive for excellence," "strive for quality," and "work hard to improve patient outcome[s]." Nurses "have good clinical skills with procedures" and "are generally knowledgeable of their craft." In addition, "nursing practice is holistic, including the family and the community." We are "hard workers," "dedicated to serving patients," and good at multitasking.

Nurses "educate our patient[s]" and "integrat[e] the patient and families in the decision-making and recovering process." We "teach the patient regarding disease process, diagnostics, and lab results." Nurses "assume responsibility for all aspects of [the] patient's well-being. We rarely say 'That's not my job.'"

One nurse responded, "Many in the front lines remember we are there for the patients, and provide patient-centered care." Another nurse summed it up:

> Nursing quality indicators and patient safety: Nursing is the primary profession taking care of patients in many healthcare settings. Nurses can spot the safety issues and develop a plan to manage the risks. When patients fall or get pressure ulcers, nursing often is looked at to identify what went wrong.

Nurses have "become the most trusted of all healthcare professionals, thus providing patients a trusted forum for questions and answers." In addition, we have "established a high level of respect and trust from consumers." Nurses "model responsibility, accountability, and trustworthiness."

Communication and Mentoring

We may not communicate as well as we should, but we are improving. The increased attention on bullying has helped to lessen the likelihood of bullying. This nurse felt that we were good at mentoring and taking care of new nurses (although, as discussed in Chapter 5, many more respondents disagreed):

> Nursing is great at precepting and mentoring new grads and students. We are used to teaching each other the ropes and take pride in sharing our knowledge with others, maybe because we all can remember being the new kid on the block.

There was acknowledgement that nurse preceptors and mentors are committed and work hard. "Nurses who have chosen to be mentors are phenomenal assets to our profession," observed one respondent.

Interprofessionalism

While we still have a way to go to work more interprofessionally, we have gotten better at it, especially concerning our communication with physicians. There is "increasing appreciation for teamwork within levels of staff as well as across disciplines." Nurses now have better relationships with physicians than we did in the past. "Relationships with other professionals, including [physicians], have improved enormously. Of course this also depends upon the attitudes of the other professionals; [it] cannot be just nursing."

We are good collaborators. One nurse respondent said, "We are the best liaisons between the patients and all the other healthcare professions." Some mentioned that the profession is "welcoming men, and not just for lifting [and] orderly duties."

Use of Ancillary Staff

We utilize ancillary staff to do things that require less education and less critical decision-making. We are good at "delegating non-nursing tasks to non-professional staff." There is a "variety of clinical rotations," and "staffing is improving."

> **NOTE**
>
> *Several chapters in this book discuss our ongoing difficulty deciding whether we want to allow the use of ancillary staff, how to best utilize them, and whether they are taking away our jobs.*

Empowerment

We have gotten better at blowing our own horns and standing up for nursing and advanced practice nursing. "We are standing up FINALLY for advanced practice nurses!" cheered one nurse respondent. We celebrate our history and work hard to control what is and should remain under the purview of nursing rather than be subsumed into other disciplines. "I think we work hard to keep control of those things that belong to nursing," noted one nurse. Nursing "controls its own destiny" and "stands behind nursing policy and practice."

Many nurse respondents celebrated our professionalism, empowerment, and adaptability. "Nurses are adaptable. As such we as a profession embrace and meet challenges faced in healthcare." They applauded our efforts to explore "advanced and expanding roles in response to societal needs." We "emphasize that we are part of a profession."

Some participants mentioned the contributions made by the profession. Nursing "focuses on things nurses can do to change their working environment for the better, at least in some places" and "encourage[s] nurses to use [the] nursing process and not blindly follow orders." We've "increased [our] voice and responsibility in hospital administration," said one nurse, and our leadership is thought by some to be improving. However, others feel that the profession "protects incompetent managers and mislabels many as leaders."

Evidence-Based Practice

Nurse respondents liked the increased emphasis on evidence-based practice (EBP), with more interest from nurses and "more access to evidence based literature." The accessibility of EBP guidelines and readable research is appreciated as nurses incorporate these into their work. We now place greater emphasis on wellness and disease prevention. One respondent observed, "Nursing professionals have the skill set needed to be able to provide preventative care and health teaching to patients in all settings."

Advocacy

We are strong patient advocates and continue to be viewed as the most trusted profession. "The general public regards nurses as a trusted profession. Nurses need to maintain professionalism to support that." We "maintain a positive image within society as a trusted profession." We are good at providing patient-centered care and at including families in our planning and education of patients. Nurses are ethical and honest, trustworthy, and visible. As one nurse said, "Nurses are consistently voted among professions with the highest integrity in the U.S.! We should continue to build upon that."

Nurses are good at "caring for people in crisis" and "caring for the whole patient" while "balanc[ing] technological and scientific aspects of nursing with the caring/healing aspects." Respondents emphasized the caring aspects of nursing, our compassion, and our dedication to providing safe, holistic care to our patients and communities. Nurses put patients and families first and place a high value on assessing and educating patients. "Nurses are generally good at helping their patients navigate the increasingly complex healthcare system."

Business and Technology

There are now more business opportunities for nurses, as well as many more options for work settings such as "pharmaceuticals, government, [and] policy preparation." Many nurse respondents praised the technology available in practice settings, such as the electronic health record and equipment that saves nursing time.

Policy

We have become more transparent in our communication about how policy changes affect nursing. Further, there appears to be increased awareness of the need to speak up and participate in health policy issues that affect us and our patients. However, nurse respondents clearly desire more input and a stronger, more united voice in nursing and health policy.

Better Pay and High Standards

One nurse noted, "Nursing has done a tremendously good job at improving our economic status. I started in the nursing field in the early 1970s and nurses' pay is much higher up the scale than it used to be." The profession "continually works to develop working conditions that are attractive and optimal for RNs." However, as will be discussed in Chapter 5, pay for both nurse educators and clinicians requires review.

The profession has high standards for practice and quality. "Workplaces have policies and procedures in place for clear definition of what can and can't be done." Several nurses praised the magnet designation: "Magnet hospitals [include] a great deal of nursing input about operations."

Nurse respondents felt that the profession has made strides in expanding nursing leadership. Several praised the efforts of the American Nurses Association (ANA). One nurse said:

> I know that ANA and NLN work hard to represent nursing in healthcare policy talks…however, I don't really know as much as I'd like to know about this, and I'm SURE that the general public has NO IDEA that nursing is involved in this way because it's never talked about in the news.

Many more nurses discussed the lack of unity among nursing organizations as a hindrance to advancing nursing's agenda.

We Are Excellent Advocates and Educators

Nurses are generally good at helping their patients navigate the increasingly complex healthcare system. We develop and support "health promotion programs" and "focus on prevention of disease instead of treatment of disease." Nurses are excellent patient educators and advocates. "Educat[ing] patients and families in the community care setting," "educat[ing] the youth as well as older consumers [about] available resources to maintain health," and "educat[ing] patients…to making wise healthcare choices." We know that "educating consumers… makes good economic sense."

"Nursing is nonpartisan. Nurses are able to advocate for all patients." In addition, we "provide an opportunity for increased access to care"—particularly to primary care—"by promoting [the] role of [the] NP." We help people access "affordable insurance and [we] broaden preventive care" by "encourag[ing] [the]uninsured and underinsured to use low-cost or free clinic services."

We Have Gained Ground for APRNs

Nursing has had some success in "advancing nursing responsibilities" so that "advanced practice nurses have become recognized as valuable in the healthcare system." One nurse said, "I believe that our nurses in the advanced role are taking the challenge to medicine by opening their own practices and YES, being team leaders in the clinics." Another added: "APRNs are stepping up to the plate to fill in for the physician shortages that are beginning to impact the healthcare system."

Many nurse participants praised the role of the APRN, their scope of practice, their high-quality outcomes, and their "excellent credentials to provide quality care to patients." APRNs are more visible in primary care, in rural settings, and with underserved populations. There is increased autonomy for APRNs, which has led to increased quality and cost-effectiveness.

Most Trusted Profession

The public recognizes that the "role of [the] RN is essential in care." Nursing is the "most trusted profession" because we "communicate well with consumers of care," make the "client's needs paramount," provide "service to those in need," "support change for patient welfare," and "respect patient autonomy in decision-making."

Another nurse proudly commented, "I believe that WE NURSES have helped frame the U.S. healthcare policy...with our good, safe practices and patient satisfaction." Others wrote of our ability to "deliver quality evidence-based care," "compassionate care," "safe, effective care," and "patient-centered" high-quality care.

We Work Well in Teams

Nurses are proud that the profession is "promoting interprofessional teamwork" and that there is renewed and "increased emphasis on inter-professional clinical teamwork" without taking an "anti-physician stance." We have made targeted "attempts to insert nursing as a player with a seat at the table." One nurse observed, "By focusing on quality care, nurses can be perceived as powerful members of the healthcare team."

Home and Community Health

"Schools of nursing are [focusing] more [on] public health" and on "work in rural areas." We "support community health initiatives." Many nurses feel that home and community health nursing work is finally getting well-deserved visibility. "Nurses are leaders in the home health and community health environment," noted one nurse. Several commented on changes that have occurred in home and community health settings: "Home healthcare has improved in the past few years," and "home health is offered to those who need it." There is "increased use of home health and community health."

Openness and Fairness

The profession appears "open to consider[ing] new ways of doing things to meet changing societal needs and expectations." It also appears to have the "flexibility to adapt to changes." "Nurses are willing to provide resource[s], research, and evidence to support health policy," observed one respondent. "Nurses have the mind-set to plan and evaluate programs effectively" and to "challenge the status quo."

Survey respondents cite the profession's support of "affordable insurance and broader preventive care," and increased access to care through the role of the nurse practitioner, free clinics, and increased cost consciousness. One nurse said, "We don't see color or financial status when treating our patients. Even though we are aware of the differences." Another said, "Nursing does not want to make care decisions based on health insurance. They want to treat all that need it the same."

Affordable Care Act

Regarding the Affordable Care Act (ACA), one nurse commented, "Nursing has long been asking for and advocating for healthcare reform so that all can have affordable medical care." Nurses are instrumental in educating the public about the ACA and "attempting to get accurate information out to the public and to the nurses on how the ACA affects the ability to provide care." One nurse noted:

> Professional associations provide the opportunity for nurses to actively participate in governmental policy-making committees by appointment so that a variety of background experiences are brought forth for consideration in the planning and execution of the various ACA programs.

Some nurses feel that "we are the reason that [the] ACA will be successful," while others worry that "not enough information [is] given to nurses to pass on to patients."

Lobbying

"Nurses serve as 'witnesses' in public to speak out for important topics," noted one nurse. According to another, however, "We are involved (but not enough)." We have made good use of the "IOM 'Future of Nursing Report' to make nurses more visible" and "increase[d] our presence in healthcare policy."

Nurses make good lobbyists in both the informal and formal meanings of the word. "Nursing is involved in lobbying for multistate licensure and practicing without limitations on a state-by-state basis" and in lobbying for better patient-nurse ratios and "better reimbursement to APNs."

"Most educated nurses are involved in small numbers in healthcare policy lobbying, testifying, etc." Many respondents commented on lobbying efforts by nurses and the increased involvement of "ordinary" nurses in efforts to change policy. "Nursing is visible to policy makers," said one nurse. The increased visibility of nursing to the public and policy makers was clearly an issue of importance to survey respondents.

One nurse commented that the "American Academy of Nurse Practitioners [and the] American College [of] Nurse Practitioners [had] united for one voice." Others praised the efforts of nursing organizations to stay on top of current issues and inform their membership about them. One mentioned that "state and national professional organizations [are] watchdogs."

Conclusion

Clearly, nurses think that as a profession, we are doing many things well. We provide several classes to students that prepare them well to pass the state board exams. We have built-in flexibility of educational pathways—perhaps too much. (This is discussed in Chapter 5.) However, we do seem to recognize the need to learn and appreciate research, evidence-based practice, and scholarship. Nursing education has increased its focus to include the needs of veterans and an emphasis on diversity and cultural sensitivity. There has been some improvement in clinical experiences for students, particularly with the advent of nurse residencies. Nurses appreciate preceptors and faculty who are current clinically and who are devoted to student success.

The nursing profession is supportive of innovation and the use of technology to care for patients. We pride ourselves on providing high-quality, safe, and ethical care, and in being the most trusted profession. We are the best patient advocates. We have worked hard to improve the physician-nurse relationship and to build interprofessional collaboration. We encourage lifelong learning, continuing education, and nurse involvement in healthcare policy and lobbying efforts. APRNs have made significant strides, and nurses seem to roundly support their success and future endeavors.

I agree that we have many things about which we should be justly proud. The following box lists aspects of the profession that nurse respondents identified as our successes. However, within the arenas of education, practice, and policy, there are other aspects in which we have been less successful. Chapter 5 discusses the responses from the great majority of respondents who strongly emphasized their concerns about where we are and where we are going.

PRIMARY POSITIVE ASPECTS

NURSING EDUCATION

Multiple pathways and program variety

Excellent courses

Specialization programs

Improvements in clinical experiences

Dedication of educators

Innovation

NURSING PRACTICE

Continuing education

Quality care

Communication and mentoring

Interprofessionalism

Use of ancillary staff

Empowerment

Evidence-based practice

Advocacy

Business and technology

POLICY

Better pay and higher standards

Advocacy

Gained ground for APRNs

Trusted

Teamwork

Community and home health

Openness and fairness

Lobbying efforts

Chapter 5
What Are We Doing Wrong?

"It's fatal 100% of the time, and he is a hospice admission anyway, so we can't just take care of him ourselves," I said. "I'll call Carol at hospice and tell them that their new patient, Mr. Hargrove, has arrived in our nursing home from New York City." I continued, "He's probably one of the only cases in America right now. I'll have someone call the Centers for Disease Control and ask them to fax some information to us about the disease and the nursing care while we admit him."

Boyish looking and tanned, Tom Hargrove, a 46-year-old math teacher, lay unconscious on the gurney at the nurses' station. His wife stood by him and murmured soothing comments. Mr. Hargrove was decerebrate and unconscious. Incredibly, the information sent by the CDC was minimal. It was accompanied by a recent publication entitled "Creutzfeldt-Jakob Disease." I scanned its contents and read and reread the sentence: "all body fluids are contaminated with the prion that causes this disease."

With barely any guidance to go on, we placed Mr. Hargrove in a private room next to the nurses' station while our staff set up an isolation room. I called in the staff and explained the situation, allayed fears, and instructed everyone to care for Mr. Hargrove using strict isolation precautions. Working in tandem with the hospice nurses, we would give our special patient the best care possible. He was our sleeping beauty, a visitor to our nursing home who challenged all our senses and professional skill.

Mr. Hargrove was with us for 5 months. Making rounds on Christmas morning, I passed his room on the way to see another patient, intending to return when I finished my rounds. But 30 years of nursing experience pulled me as though magnetized into his room. He had ceased to breathe. We prepared his body according to the strict instructions we had been given. We all shed tears of pride because Tom's skin had remained intact and we had protected ourselves and everyone in the nursing home from contamination.

Chapter 4, "What Are We Doing Right?" described what surveyed nurses considered positive aspects of nursing today. This chapter uses their words to illustrate the problems they encounter on a daily basis and the concerns they have with regard to education, practice, and policy.

Education

Chapter 4, "What Are We Doing Right?," discussed what nurse respondents liked about nursing education. Nevertheless, there are several aspects of how we educate new and graduate nurses that perturbed and disturbed them. Many of the issues that concerned them are not new. Indeed, they hearken back to what was discussed in Chapter 1, "Nurses Are Made Not Born: Educational Reform Frames the Profession (1900–1935)," Chapter 2, " Rising from the Depths: We Are Not Subservient (1935-1970)," and Chapter 3, "Clinicians, Scientists, and Scholars: Separate but Equal (1970–2000)."

Multiple Pathways and Program Variety

While some nurses in Chapter 4 praised the flexibility of multiple pathways to enter practice, others think that "multiple pathways into the profession hinder a strong standard and nursing's recognition by other professions." The survey confirmed that the debate about entry level to practice is tremendously controversial. One nurse wrote:

> Educational programs for entering nursing are inconsistent. This fragments nursing education and dilutes the argument that nursing is a profession that should have the same respect as pharmacists, physical therapists, doctors, engineers, [and] lawyers. For example, the LVN [licensed vocational nurse] to RN programs, ADN [associate degree in nursing] to MSN [master's of science in nursing], MEL [master's entry level programs for initial entry]…Some programs require RNs to have a BSN to enter advanced nursing programs, others require three to six classes to bridge into a masters, others accept an ADN with a BA [bachelor of arts]/BS [bachelor of science] in another discipline to enter an MSN [program]. These programs have surely provided access to nursing and degree advancement, and were needed to address the shortage, but [they] have also fragmented perceptions of nurses, not only by the general public but by other occupations mentioned above. We should be viewed as equal to other established professional careers.

While the majority of survey respondents recommend enforcing the BSN as entry into the profession, many propose equivalent clinical time and opportunities for real-life preparation as provided in non-BSN nursing programs. (See Chapter 6 for further discussion on this.)

> We need one entry into practice level! BSN. AS [associate degree in science] and [the] diploma no longer serve our needs. Too many AS graduates are disappointed when they cannot find work. Also, this tends to confuse the clients. What is the difference between the AS and BS nurse? Why do other professions have higher entry levels? Nursing needs to come to a final decision on this: BSN as entry level, MSN for management, and DNP [doctor of nursing practice] or PhD for our leaders and nurse practitioners.

Another nurse said:

> The allowance of poorly accredited and poor-scoring ADN and certification schools just to "meet nursing demands" lowers the value of the profession. As nurses, we

> need to rally to remove existence of such programs to el-
> evate our profession and keep patients safe. The nursing
> product should remain consistent.

Several respondents, however, expressed concern and anger about
requiring the BSN and see it as a reflection on nurses with ADNs or
diplomas, judging them to be somehow inferior and

> creating dissension among the profession. We are our
> own worst enemy, doing away with LPNs [licensed prac-
> tical nurse] and now treating ADN's as though they are
> the LPNs of the past, when a BSN and ADN take the
> same nursing test to practice nursing.

Many ask that these options continue to exist to enable people who
cannot afford 4 years of college to become nurses. Others complain that
the profession

> has not provided for effective transition to BSN programs
> from other degrees. Currently an AD grad need only take
> four nursing courses, and then a host of credits in the
> "electives," which does not adequately prepare nurses for
> professional nursing practice.

Some suggested implementing different levels of licensure and
certification as an alternative to requiring the BSN.

> Nursing is pushing nurses to go from AD (sometimes on-
> line) to BS to MS and DNP [with] no identification to
> nursing there. Real nursing needs to come from establish-
> ing nursing as your profession...The best nurses I have
> ever met were diploma nurses that grew up the ladder as
> a nurse.

In an effort to get nurses through our programs, we often engage
in "too much spoon-feeding. Students do not take responsibility for
learning." Others expressed dissatisfaction with the accelerated programs
that allow non-nurses to enter programs that lead directly to the nurse
practitioner certification either by way of the MSN or DNP. They contend
that the RN needs 3 to 5 years of experience before entering any nurse
practitioner (NP) program to be effective and to practice efficiently and
safely.

Several respondents took issue with the increasing use of online programs to educate nurses; "distance learning programs for NPs... cannot prepare students effectively." Many respondents objected to the need to acquire a DNP. One respondent stated that the DNP is being "jammed down the throats" of NPs and that this should stop. One survey respondent noted:

> Nursing continues to keep mandating higher level[s] of education for certain nursing practices. For example, the need for DNP as entry-level education into [the] nurse practitioner role. Nursing can be our own worst enemy in advancing the nursing profession.

Others report that there is no place for a nurse with a DNP. One nurse said, "Nursing has not created room for DNPs to practice. The expectation is for the entry level to be DNP, yet DNP-prepared nurses have to teach or stay in their previous positions." Another nurse remarked that students who move straight through the BSN to DNP may not have the wherewithal to do what is expected of them in DNP programs:

> [I'm] skeptical about the clinical preparation of the BSN to DNP. [I] am keeping an open mind but feel that the paradigm of preparation reflects more that of medical students. Quite frankly, I don't see how an FNP [family nurse practitioner] that has never practiced can identify a contemporary practice issue in their workplace. [I] am keeping an open mind, though, and will see how the graduates of this new degree perform clinically.

Some respondents feel that we admit students who have no chance of graduating. One nurse observed:

> ADN programs are enrolling many students, many of whom have no hope of graduating. More screening should be done to ensure that those entering the program of study will be successful.

This may be true for BSN programs as well, although admission to BSN programs tends to be highly competitive. Others think that there should be less emphasis on grades and more emphasis on other factors. One nurse noted, "[There is] acceptance to program[s] primarily based on prerequisite grades. Life experience should be considered more."

This is a growing trend, especially with regard to military veterans who are increasingly being given college credit for their military experience.

Interestingly, more respondents commented on the increasing tendency to admit students who are not qualified and to see them through to graduation than they did on neglecting to admit students who should be given a chance to get a nursing education. "All programs must ensure that their foreign students are fluent in English before they are placed in clinical settings." Another nurse said, "Protect [nursing] from intellectually challenged nursing students." Another went further: "Screen applicants for acceptance in regards to character, periodic drug screens, past job performance, criminal history, honesty." Poor writing skills are also of concern and inhibit recognition as professionals.

Nurse Educators

Nurses take issue with a number of aspects of the educator role, ranging from inadequate pay, to poor preparation for the role, to insufficient numbers of nurse educators to prepare graduates well. We are "not paying faculty at a level that attracts the best and the brightest early in their careers." In addition, there is "poor communication and collaboration between nursing educators and nursing clinicians" and "the profession does not transition new nurses or new nurse educators or nurse scientists well."

The lack of or insufficient faculty practice continues to undermine the ability of faculty to provide instruction about what's current clinically. "Instructors may have the educational requirements but are not always the most skilled in practice." One nurse noted:

> Perhaps most importantly, we do not honor the work that goes into educating nurses and as such the pay for faculty is terrible. It is nearly impossible to recruit good faculty into our programs. Why would any sane person leave a hospital management job or a bedside nursing position where you can make 50% more? It's very difficult...securing someone with the proper credentials is yet another confounding factor.

According to one nurse, we should "mentor excellent faculty. Many faculty are simply graduates of the programs in which they teach and are not expert educators." Another nurse commented, "Train nurse educators to be nurse educators and routinely assign mentors until they become proficient."

Insufficient and Inadequate Clinical Preparation

There seems to be overwhelming concern that nurse educators, both in the classroom and in clinical settings, are not experientially prepared to teach students clinical practice. Further, it is misguided to assume that staff nurses with clinical experience are excellent teachers. Our need for more nurse educators has been the impetus for taking "warm bodies" into nursing education.

Many nurses expressed anger that being a bedside nurse is not considered "enough," and that the lack of adequate, real-life clinical preparation while in school is ignored because it is taken for granted that graduates will quickly move away from the bedside. Along these same lines, some expressed concern that students are learning too much about health policy and not enough about how to take care of the patient and meet the patient's basic needs. "Teach time management and compassion," noted one respondent. Several recommend increasing opportunities for simulation experiences while in school, but only to hone skills that need to be used in the clinical setting, not as a substitute for taking care of real patients.

The comments and concerns about clinical preparation were so numerous and adamant among the survey responses that it is worth listing the primary themes and some exemplars:

- **Lack of preparation for the real world:**

  [There is a] "lack of connection to practice in nursing education. As someone who is in both practice and education, I feel like they are preparing nurses for a world that doesn't exist."

  [There is a] "failure to prepare nurses for the bedside experience."

- **Insufficient quality:**

  [There is a] "lessening quality of [the] clinical experience leading to graduates who are not clinically competent."

  [There is] "not enough actual hands-on experience—that is, clinical work."

- **Back to the basics:**

  [Students] "need more exposure to basic nursing skills, listening."

  [There is] "not enough emphasis on the ritual of the bath, mouth care, [and] back rubs, which people really respond to in healing."

  "Actual assessment of [the] patient [is lacking]. [We need to get] back to [the] basics of caring and compassion. I was hospitalized a few years ago for several days and only one RN actually put their hands on me to assess me and to give me a back rub."

- **Insufficient clinical hours:**

  [There are] "not enough clinical hours to prepare the student for real time."

- **Time management:**

  "Having one patient as a nursing student and then being assigned six or more as a new nurse" [does not prepare the student to manage their time].

- **Clinical reasoning:**

  [Students don't understand the] "clinical/scientific under-pinnings of practice."

- **Too much simulation:**

  [There is] "too much time in simulation settings."

- **Socialization into the profession:**

  "New nurses need to be better prepared for things like the socialization process of becoming a new nurse."

- **Poor preparation of clinical faculty:**

   "Prepare adjunct faculty to be efficient in providing excellent education in the clinical setting."

- **Exposure to various settings:**

   [We should be] "thinking outside the box on clinical placements and helping [students] understand these are real places nurses work."

   "Provide meaningful and increasingly more involved clinical education in a variety of settings."

Cost and Career

Several respondents commented on the cost of a nursing education, saying it is prohibitive and a barrier to progressing through school. One nurse noted, "Most programs are too expensive for many potential nurses." Another was more specific: "We support more foreign nursing students with scholarships and financial aid, rather [than] local/national students who stay and impact the local workforces." The profession could also do more with regard to career planning, assisting new graduates to find jobs, and helping them "transition to professional practice."

Research and Critical Thinking

Several respondents lamented that there is not enough emphasis on the ability to critically evaluate research or to think critically in general. Views are mixed with regard to the value of learning nursing theory, but many agree that there is not enough emphasis placed on the foundations of nursing, conceptual underpinnings, systems thinking, prioritization, and basic common sense. One nurse commented:

   Basic nursing 101 has been lost. Nurses used to be critical thinkers who could examine a problem and devise a plan of care to help. Critical thinking has decreased among nurses at the bedside. I am [a] wound ostomy continence specialist. I often am called to see patients with severe incontinence dermatitis. The male patient may be incontinent of urine that could easily be contained with a condom catheter. Why is it I am the first person to suggest [this]? Because the nurse is not thinking.

Practice

Many of the concerns about nursing education naturally overlap with concerns about what occurs in nursing practice. This is because nurses tend to bring to practice what they have been taught in school.

Disunity Continues

Many nurses responded vehemently about the inability of nurses to work together and speak with one voice. As one nurse noted, there is

> too much fragmentation—we think of ourselves as IV [intravenous] nurses, OR [operating room] nurses, pedi[atric] nurses, etc., rather than [as] "nurses," and our professional organizations generally follow suit. This makes it hard to have a unified voice represent us as a whole.

Basics of Care

Nurses complain that new graduates don't always understand the basics of patient care from assessment to simple ways of caring. Spending time with patients, being less dependent on machines to assess and care for the patient, and using listening techniques to interact with family members are skills that are rapidly being lost.

On the subject of patient care, one nurse noted:

> Twelve-hour shifts may be good for nurses and their personal lives, but it has been at the expense of patient care. There is such a lack of continuity in hospitals and other areas that have the 12-hour shift. Some units, such as PACU, ambulatory surgery, or OR/endoscopy, can do 12-hour shifts because the patient schedule differs daily. But inpatient units should have 8-hour shifts or at the least a 10-hour, 4-day work week. I cannot tell you how

frustrating it is to hear "I don't know, it is my first day with this patient." The nurses rarely work back-to-back days, so the patient suffers with different nurses each day and night. This creates a situation where subtle signs may be missed because the nurse on duty is not aware that it is new and does not report [it]. Also, I feel the 12-hour shift fosters the "working [to buy] that refrigerator" attitude. The nurse, if putting in her 12 hours, could care less what happens to the patient the next day. Sad but true.

It is interesting that this nurse's comments echo those of nurses in the 1920s, when the profession worked so hard to cut working hours from 12 hours to 8 hours.

Poor Transition of New Graduates

There is overwhelming interest in standardizing and requiring internships, mentorships, and residencies for new nursing graduates. Practicing nurses feel that new graduates need standardized programs to help them acclimate to their work environments and to be less burdensome on their colleagues as they learn their duties. Recent graduates from diploma, associate degree, bachelor's degree, and master's degree programs confirmed that they, too, marvel at the disparity in length, breadth, and depth of orientations and precepted opportunities and feel that they and their colleagues suffer because of it (Neal-Boylan, 2013).

It is not uncommon for new graduates from associate degree programs (who are not typically offered classes in leadership) and BSN programs to be put into positions of leadership before they have become the least bit comfortable in their role as a nurse. Leadership is a fundamental component of the BSN curriculum. However, content may vary across schools, and students may not be learning enough about the realities of leadership before graduation. These new graduates typically do not receive orientations or mentoring regarding how to perform their leadership duties. One nurse respondent observed, "Mentoring of new nurses continues to be viewed as inadequate by many nurses, with few opportunities for residencies."

Survey respondents support formal training of preceptors and a lengthy period of time in which new graduates, whether from an undergraduate or a graduate program, can practice in an environment in which they can safely make mistakes and learn how to be nurses or how to practice in a new nursing role.

In general, "graduate learning is very independent with little positive reinforcement during the process." Nurse practitioner students are not always prepared for the reality of practice because "NPs are not prepared to provide quality care without strong support systems." Students need to learn how to be leaders, to delegate, and to prevent and resolve conflicts so they are prepared to function as nurses in real practice.

Finding Jobs

"Academics prepare nurses to fill the ideal jobs that don't exist for 90% of new grads. Real-world shock results." New graduates are not sufficiently encouraged to seek jobs outside of acute care. Those nurses who get jobs outside of the traditional hospital setting don't always receive the respect they deserve. There is "continued lack of respect for those nurses in alternative settings, as in corrections, parole or probation offices, community clinics, and doing home visits in very challenging areas."

In my work with nurses with disabilities, I have discovered that although many of these nurses are pushed out of hospital jobs because of unfounded concerns that they will jeopardize patient safety, some eventually find jobs in non-hospital settings and are quite content. Many would not have considered these jobs, or even been aware of them, had they not been forced to leave the hospital setting. However, they expressed high job satisfaction. Their physical disabilities did not affect their ability to perform the job, and they felt valued for their expertise rather than judged for their disability. It is important that student nurses and nurses in general be made more aware of the opportunities and challenges of non-hospital settings and of the fact that nurses can have tremendous impact in these settings.

Difficulty Working With Others

One nurse noted that although we've made some progress, we should:

> Encourage nursing training with medical students. In the real world, nurses and doctors interact frequently. This

was never practiced in nursing school. [It would be good] to have a course where nursing students and medical students work together; we should encourage interdisciplinary care.

The need to improve communication skills with people of other disciplines was cited frequently, as were diversity training and the need to learn coping techniques to manage within an environment in which bullying is prevalent. As observed by one nurse:

> The nursing management does not want to deal with lateral workplace violence. ([There is] no education about it.) Management enforces smiles to patients, but ignores the needs of nurses or of those bullied. [Bullies] try to get other nurses to do their work, they lie, they manipulate. There is a lack of ethics across all disciplines.

Incivility and bullying were common themes among the responses to the survey. Although the profession has acknowledged these problems, clearly there is much work still to be done to eliminate them.

We do not model self-care or good health. "New nurses need to know about how to take good care of themselves in terms of self-care. Moral distress, burnout, and compassion fatigue are all real issues." We need to do more to "promote nurse wellness."

There is still a strong perception that nurses eat their young. "Many nurses working in the clinical settings are still not welcoming to students," said one nurse. Another nurse said, "Older nurses have forgotten that they once were a student and are not always gracious to help students learn." We are not good at taking care of each other. "We fight among ourselves and degrade others in our profession. We value some types of nursing more than others."

The ability to communicate appropriately and effectively continues to be a problem once nurses begin to practice. One nurse noted that we should "have productive conversations with colleagues" and "rise to the level of colleague versus subordinate to physicians. This is an attitude, not a role." Many nurse respondents commented about ongoing problems communicating with physicians and feeling undervalued. "Relationships between the disciplines still are not where they should be."

One nurse decried the "degrading, humiliating, or insulting clinicians when there is a questionable order or plan of care. We forget most facilities are teaching ones and that a doctor is someone who simply graduated medical school."

The Push to Return to School

Several nurses think the push for higher education discourages nurses from staying at the bedside or thinking of bedside nursing as valuable. According to one nurse, it "makes new grads think being a floor nurse is a temporary job. So many new grads state they just want a few years experience (or do none at all) before starting NP programs." Another nurse said that there are "too many applicants to nursing programs for the job security. We have to have caregivers invested in health and wellness." Moreover, "Some of the students are there to ace the program, but not to take care of patients ([they are] headed for a desk job). [It's a] means to an end and better pay."

There is a lack of attention to how to behave at the bedside and how to give comprehensive quality care to fulfill basic patient and family needs. "[There is] not enough training on the importance of being present" with the patient. "Not enough on being with the dying" and "not enough time at the actual bedside with family interaction." Another commented, "A lot of the younger nursing professionals currently graduating are in it for the money and not the patient care; priorities on patient care are not being promoted." Discharge planning may also suffer:

> [The] patient [is] admitted, [the] RN knows [the] diagnosis, but does not have or does not take the thought process other than task completion and charting. They need to look at the total picture. Management doesn't assist in this thought process at my current [place of] employment.

Many expressed that the push to obtain a graduate degree sacrifices quality care by "allowing students to matriculate through from baccalaureate to PhD with no practical experience of being a nurse, especially if their goal is to teach nursing."

Lack of Professionalism

"In [the] past decade I have noted a distinct lack of professionalism," noted one nurse. "New grads have more unprofessional attitudes— arrogance. They don't know what they don't know." Nurses echoed the sentiments of several respondents, who believe that we should "encourage accountability, work ethic, and professionalism." There's "still too much infighting on [an] organizational level and between specialties."

Utilization of Unlicensed Personnel

While a few respondents stated that unlicensed personnel should be utilized more often in clinical settings, the majority were troubled by their overuse and lack of preparation to do what was expected of them. They cited "too much reliance on unlicensed assistive personnel" and "allowing the use of medical assistants without competency requirements." Nurses are concerned that "medical assistants [MAs] are not a substitute for RNs, yet facilities utilize MAs over RNs." The original intention to use unlicensed personnel to assist the nurse "did not accomplish the goal[s] of reducing RN workload and improv[ing] patient safety."

Policy

Nurses expressed strong feelings about our inability to present a collective voice with regard to policy and the need to improve our public image.

Disunity

"We do not use our collective voice (which could be very powerful)." Many nurses responded that they don't feel well-prepared to engage in policy discussions or to advocate for the profession in the policy arena. "The role of public health/preventative health is under emphasized, [as are] disaster management, community engagement, etc." One nurse recommended that we "teach nurses about public policy and how it directly affects patient care and the healthcare system overall." Nurses ask that the profession "encourage civic engagement," "encourage active participation in political realms," and "promote membership in our national professional association."

The perception that we are not good at joining with one another to speak in one voice is pervasive. One nurse said, "We don't protect one another or enable all nurses to join our organizations so they can feel supported and provide support to colleagues." Another commented. "Professional nursing associations are too expensive and theoretical. This discourages first line nurses from joining."

The theme of disunity reappears in survey responses pertaining to education, practice, and policy, and much of its cause has to do with cost. Another major cause is perceived elitism, which is discussed in more detail throughout the rest of this book.

Poor Understanding of Business, Economics, Governance, and Finance

Many nurses don't understand the economics or business side of nursing and healthcare, and appreciate that this deficiency may hold them back. As one nurse put it, there is "not enough [time] devoted to [the] business side of healthcare." Students have "no exposure to healthcare finance courses" and schools are "lacking content on health economics and value."

Another nurse suggested, "I think we could do better in encouraging student nurses and graduate nurses to be part of solutions by becoming active either in the ANA or shared governance programs. The word 'politics' needs to stop being seen as a dirty word."

Leaders Who Are Ineffective and Not Grounded in Reality

The distance of many nurse leaders from the reality of nursing is a concern. One nurse noted, "ANA, members of nursing's elite, and top educators [are] not in touch with reality." There seems to be a perception among some nurses that the "ANA has not formally advocated for collegiate nursing education since 1965."

Nursing leaders may make decisions for their organizations or the profession as a whole without the context of recent clinical practice experience. One nurse observed, "Nursing leaders often have no recent clinical experience. Some ideas are unrealistic." In addition, nurses, both in academe and in clinical practice, want to move away from transactional leadership models to those employing transformational leadership techniques. They are not satisfied with "nursing leaders such as CNOs [chief nursing officers] who are not transformational."

Nurses report that healthcare is "too dominated by physicians and administrators" and that the "lack of commitment by management (hospital) impacts nursing attitude[s] and practice in a negative way." There are "top-down policies designed by management with no sense of day-to-day, hour-to-hour pressures." In addition, physicians should be kept out of decisions about nursing practice.

Hospital administrators place a heavy burden on nurses by adding "tasks...to nursing assignments that do nothing for patient care." In addition, "upper management sends down the heavy hand to change [but] no one to support and pat the lower staff on the head to say they did a good job."

Nurses who are paid hourly are not always treated with the respect due to professionals, while administrators put "nurses into management positions by default with no management skills." Nurses should "stand up against management that are making poor decisions." One nurse commented, "We don't advocate for ourselves in healthcare facilities; we let others make decisions that negatively impact our practice and patient care."

Nurses are not always utilized to the highest degree of their education or ability and do not work autonomously, even when they are capable of doing so and licensed as such. Nurses are overburdened and overworked. "Nurses work beyond their scheduled hours, while off the clock—there are unreasonable expectations about how much we can do."

Nurses commented that there is too much gossip and too much time wasted on non-nursing activities. In addition, there is inadequate time to give medications correctly, attend to patients' spiritual needs, make appropriate referrals to hospice and palliative care, or treat patient pain adequately or appropriately. "Too many tasks [are] placed on floor nurses. [There are] increased responsibilities and tasks per patient with computerized charting and barcode medication administration systems."

Lack of Professional Image

We have not been successful in demonstrating our full value. As one nurse wrote:

> [Nursing] has never been able to raise the level of prestige of the profession. ([I] believe this is due to having the lowest requirements for education to enter practice.) We have respect as a profession, but not prestige, and prestige is, for better or worse, what attracts young people to any profession.

Nurses still feel that there are many misconceptions about what nurses do, partly because we keep changing the rules. "The public and other health professionals are not always clear on our various roles, titles, and associated responsibilities, discrediting who we are as a professional body."

One nurse said, "We do not do a good job of explaining what is nursing and what isn't, what makes us different from the CNA [certified nurse's aide]. Everyone in the doctor's office that isn't the doctor is called 'nurse.'" This sentiment was echoed by many other survey participants, one of whom observed, "We haven't yet sufficiently let the public in on what we do and how we do it, and how that contributes to the nation's health."

In the view of nurse respondents, we are not affecting healthcare policy as much as we'd like to. We are "not raising public awareness of what we are capable of doing, thus losing that opportunity to have more voices demanding change from lawmakers."

Contributors to this problem are that we have an "inadequate media presence" and we "make most of what nurses do invisible by letting other professions take the credit." Also, "nurses are becoming nurses for the job, not the profession, and those who should not be nurses are hurting the image of nurses."

Conclusion

While nurses commented on things we are doing well (as discussed in Chapter 4), many more raised issues and problems that require some resolution. It is well known that people who respond to self-report surveys often do so because they are anxious to voice complaints rather than make positive comments. However, nurses' concerns take on greater significance when we consider that many of these concerns have existed, in some form or another, since the birth of the profession.

The next chapter describes possible solutions raised by nurse respondents. Many are cogent, realistic, and doable. One can't help but wonder if our professional organizations were less fragmented and our conferences and journals less costly, whether suggested solutions from nurses who otherwise do not have much of a voice could help resolve many of our issues once and for all.

PRIMARY ISSUES

Fragmented education

Accelerated and online programs that may sacrifice quality

Insufficient and unqualified faculty

Disunity continues

Lack of adequate clinical preparation for new nurses

High cost of nursing education

Lack of adequate career planning

Insufficient emphasis on research and critical thinking

Need to get back to basics of nursing care

Poor transition of new graduates

Difficulties working with others

Lack of professionalism

Push to return to school

Utilization of unlicensed personnel

Disunity

continues

> *Poor understanding of business, economics, finance, and governance*
>
> *Leaders who are ineffective and are not grounded in reality*
>
> *Lack of professional image*

Reference

Neal-Boylan, L. (2013). *The nurse's reality gap: Overcoming barriers between academic achievement and clinical success*. Indianapolis, IN: Sigma Theta Tau Publishing.

Chapter 6

Nurses Propose Solutions to Education, Practice, and Policy Issues

It was my anxiety at being in the OR, not being a selectively listening 19-year-old student. Some people think it's a magical place, the OR, but it's hot and confining and sterile.

I know the procedures now; it's the second time I have been assigned to the OR. I can't very well tell our instructor that I hate the heat and the running in and out of the OR theater for supplies when ordered to do so by the surgeon or resident. That is the job of the circulating nurse, after all. It's 1951, and our second year of nursing school. They have expectations of us now. We can't put flowers in the urinal as we did when we were "probies," I tell myself as I run to central supply for more retractors. Will I find them? Heck, I can read labels on the shelves, but they said to hurry, and I do so. I find the correct package in its muslin wrap. There is a strip label on each package with the date and hour the instrument was autoclaved for sterilization by the central supply staff.

It's some sort of abdominal case, I see as I return to the OR. I hand the package, which I have carefully and correctly (as taught) unwrapped without breaking sterility, to give to the

OR nurse. The OR nurse is a graduate. She is quiet, standing opposite the surgeon. Her movements are spare, precise, and automatic. She hands him each instrument quickly and with grace, no words required. I know that she is beautiful underneath the cap and gown and mask. She does not appear to perspire, but the eminent Dr. Voorhees does. Clement (Dr. Cantrell), the intern, doing surgical rotation, gingerly attempts to wipe the surgeon's brow with gauze, trying not to disturb the surgeon's field of vision.

The surgical resident is Dr. Brynner. He is 6 feet 4 inches tall with tortoise-shell glasses and a shock of blond hair under his OR cap. This is probably not a good choice as a residency, I muse. Dan Brynner, bent at the waist, must accommodate Dr. Voorhees, who is about 5 feet 6 inches in his BVDs. Which one of us is dating Dan now, I wondered. Oh, it's Eileen. She will get a kick out of this picture, I think to myself as I await the next garbled order to retrieve some equipment from central supply.

As though on cue, Dr. Brynner asks me for something, mumbling through his surgical mask. I look at him and run to central supply. I haven't quite heard him or understood what he asked for, but I feel confident that central supply will have it and I will know it when I see it. I stop short in the brightly lit stockroom with all the equipment I know to be sparkling and sterile beneath muslin wrapping. The supply attendant is not there. I am alone now, with the realization that I do understand Dr. Brynner's request. I cannot fulfill his request, however, and know that I must return to the OR and "take my medicine." Indeed, when I return, they are all laughing (over the sterile field). Dr. Brynner requested "a hole to stand in," and I had dutifully tried to comply.

This chapter resounds with the actual voices of nurses who took advantage of the opportunity to offer solutions to critical and ongoing issues in nursing. There were several common themes among their responses. With regard to nursing education, most respondents agreed that the BSN should be the entry-level degree, that new nurses need strong mentoring, that education should be more standardized, that students should learn nursing theory and research, that clinical experiences are currently inadequate to prepare new nurses for the reality of practice, and that they should have a broad general education that goes beyond nursing.

Nurse respondents had a lot to say about nursing practice, including the need to restore and improve our professional image, promote self-care and reduce burnout, pay nurses what they're worth, enhance collaboration and communication both intra- and interprofessionally, decide where we stand with regard to ancillary staff, manage nurse workloads, engage in lifelong learning, and promote leadership.

Comments about nurses and policy issues concerned the need to educate students and nurses, become more politically active, work with our nursing organizations, lobby, vote, and work to promote change. Nurses exhort us to get the word out to each other and to the public, to learn and comprehend reimbursement practices, to engage in acts of good citizenship, and to unify to accomplish our goals and increase our political strength.

Education

Nurses responding to the survey contributed their thoughts and ideas about how we can improve the delivery and effectiveness of nursing education.

Require BSN Entry Level to Practice

Most nurses seem to be in favor of the BSN as entry to practice. One nurse noted, "[The] BSN [must be the] absolute minimum for entry into practice." But some suggested that nurses continue to be allowed to obtain an associate's degree due mostly to cost concerns, before moving on to get the BSN.

The Institute of Medicine (IOM; 2010) report called for 80% of nurses to have a BSN by the year 2020. Many nurses cannot afford to go directly into 4-year colleges, and would prefer to have the option to obtain an associate's degree first and then articulate into a BSN program.

One nurse proposed, "Accept ADN [associate's degree in nursing] and diploma grads as viable options for entry into practice, with a requirement that within 10 years they must get their BSN." Another spoke for many respondents with this suggestion: "Continue to build ADN-to-BSN bridge programs. Find a way to allow the ADN path to continue to exist, since it is the only path open for many people due to [the] cost of 4-year colleges." One nurse suggested we keep the various levels but "establish separate licensure (and scope of practice) for nurses with different levels of education."

One experienced nurse was very clear: "Since before 1967 (when I started my journey), nursing has discussed the different levels of entry. [It's] time to stop 'piddle, twiddle, and resolving' and just declare the BSN as the entry level to sit for the NCLEX [nursing board exam]." Others think that the BSN does not go far enough and that we should:

> Raise the bar regarding education needed for entry into practice. I would like to see the DNP be required, but know that probably isn't realistic. I think it *is* possible to mandate at least a BSN for entry into practice like many other countries outside the U.S. have.

Even those who favor the BSN as the minimum degree are still concerned that BSN graduates do not get enough clinical time while in school. One respondent suggested, "Make sure that the BSN students are getting at least as much clinical time as their ADN and diploma peers." Another nurse said, "Require 4 years of clinical experience in BSN programs."

Another concern expressed about the mandate for the BSN is that it is an injunction against nurses who provide direct care. One nurse responded, "Stop making it seem like being a bedside nurse is 'not enough.' There is too much emphasis on encouraging RNs to move away from direct patient care." The nurse who provides direct care is essential to who we are as a profession. As suggested by one respondent, "Create a culture where the bedside RN is a valued member of the team."

Part of this issue seems to stem from the concern that pushing nurses too quickly into higher-level degrees will prevent them from internalizing the basics of nursing care. As one nurse said:

I was not a diploma-educated nurse[and] had a degree in sociology. I had to support four children, so I went the AD [associate degree] route. Give those young and older people a start by allowing them to work as a nurse, knowing what nurses do best. Then move them on to our goal of advanced practice. Today we push them too fast. Nursing needs to be first and foremost.

Another put it this way: "Nurses over the years (from diploma to advanced education) have come to our profession because they wanted to help people. Give them that chance to develop 'nursing mentality and practice' before moving them on."

Some nurses think that capstone experiences that include mentorships or residencies can help students learn how to care. As noted by one nurse:

Create a culture of care within the nursing professionals. Promoting mentorship and/or residency programs [in] the last semester of clinical…will enable and ease in transitioning from a student nurse to a professional nurse.

Mentoring

Nurses believe that there is still much work to be done to strengthen and standardize mentoring structures. No one disagrees that mentoring is necessary, but many believe that mentors should be chosen and trained carefully. As noted by one nurse, "All staff/clinicians need to be mentored in working with students in meaningful ways. This requires buy-in at all levels and by all healthcare professionals, especially agency administrators." Some feel that mentors should be reimbursed in some way ("offer working RNs an educational stipend or free tuition when mentoring nursing students in a clinical setting") and that mentorship should be a condition of re-licensure ("require a number of hours of mentoring/precepting to renew licensure").

Adjunct faculty who teach clinicals should know how to teach and mentor and in turn develop future mentors among new graduates. One respondent suggested the following:

Create learning environments with clinical adjuncts who can precept/mentor new grads (all levels) in real clinical settings so that the new grad can get good clinical experience, gain confidence, and ultimately become someone who can mentor the next generation of new nurses.

Nurses are frequently chosen arbitrarily to be preceptors or mentors. Often, there is no remuneration. In these cases, the student or new graduate is literally stuck learning from someone who isn't motivated to do a good job with them. To help mitigate this, one nurse suggested that we "get feedback from student nurses about the people they precept with. If they aren't offering positive experiences, don't assign them students."

Nurse respondents think that the development and management of nurse residencies should be a partnership between the school and the healthcare facility or agency. One nurse said, "Get involved in nurse residency models (do not leave all of it for hospitals to manage)." Another nurse noted, "Academic-industry partnerships should work to create 6-month residencies for all new grads." Nurses think that "in every clinical setting, there should be room for students, without exception. This should become routine and expected by healthcare professionals, patients, and families alike."

This is also an issue for students and new graduates from advanced practice programs. One nurse wrote:

> Educational programs for advanced nursing practice should have dedicated preceptorships. The culture of advanced practice nurses needs to change in such a way [that] the preceptors feel it is an honor to be selected as one who can teach another.

Standardize Nursing Education

Many nurses think we should "standardize curriculum," "standardize practices," "standardize the profession across the country and have different testing for each level of education," and "standardize nursing education" overall. We should also "revise the NP [nurse practitioner] curriculum."

There is a lot of concern about the lack of standardization of nursing education. This surprised me. As a nurse educator, I know that schools of nursing are required to meet NLN or CCNE accreditation standards and comply with *The Essentials of Baccalaureate Education for Professional Nursing Practice* (2008) (aacn.nche.edu), *The Essentials of Master's Education in Nursing* (2011) (aacn.nche.edu), and *The Essentials of Doctoral Education for Advanced Nursing Practice* (2006) (aacn. nche.edu). In addition, programs with nurse practitioner tracks must comply with standards put out by the National Organization of Nurse Practitioner Faculties (http://www.nonpf.org/), and schools are encouraged to incorporate QESN concepts (http://qsen.org/) in undergraduate and graduate education. Outside of those requirements, programs are intentionally given leeway to develop their own curricula. I think this is a good thing. Nursing is a profession, not a vocation. We should not be rigid in how we teach our students. In addition, it's important to consider geographical and demographical variances as we educate students to take care of the populations they serve.

Some think we should add more education about specialty areas in traditional nursing education. One nurse respondent wrote:

> For BSN degree programs, universities should offer specialty pathways for those seeking specialty roles in the acute [care] world. The BSN [student] should be able to take a semester of courses focusing on critical care if that is their desired pathway, with clinical experience associated as such. This will help offset the delay in experienced care for these vulnerable populations.

Others believe that we should do the following:

> Evaluate curriculum to establish what the knowledge baseline should be—i.e., do we cut out OB [obstetrics], peds [pediatrics], and other specialty practices from the curriculum, allowing a more specified curriculum without diminishing the quality or ability to prepare nurses who can think critically and respond appropriately? ([In other words] leave the specialties as areas that nurses would do "new grad" type residencies [in], since very few go into specialty practice right after graduation?)

Emphasize Theory and Research

While nurses are divided with regard to the value of learning nursing and other types of theories, those who proposed solutions had this to say: "As we put increasing value on the more educated nurse, we must alter curricula toward an evidenced-based program that more closely promotes nursing theory and nursing research," "allow for real clinicians to be paired in the classroom with formal educators to better connect theory to practice," and "encourage more educational theory for those wanting to teach."

Another emphasized the need to "incorporate increasingly complex practice in evaluating research as used in courses to teach evidence-based practice" and "relate clinical experiences directly with course theory with related learning objectives."

Broaden Knowledge

There is wide support for adding courses to the curriculum to better prepare nurses for the real world and to generally broaden their knowledge base to improve the image of the nurse as a professional. Respondents had many suggestions for what should be added to the curriculum. For example, one respondent wrote, "[Have] courses to include writing, reading, verbal communication, conflict management, critical thinking, delegation, responsibility, and authority." One nurse added commentary on the social issues nurses face: "Include the topic of addiction into the curriculum as it pertains to the nurses themselves."

Some comments were very specific, suggesting "requir[ing] gerontology class," "more wellness/nutrition," "case management classes [and] forensic classes," "society and gender roles," "foundation concepts in management, marketing, statistics, and healthcare organizations," and "healthcare history and the business aspect of the healthcare industry."

NOTE

Interestingly, no one proposed how to fit these additional subjects in without extending the length of nursing education.

Also supported were education and classes similar to what medical students receive. One respondent suggested schools "[include a] class in [the] analysis of medical research publications." Another nurse suggested we provide "advanced levels of knowledge about pathophysiology and disease processes to the level medicine learns it."

"The ACA [Affordable Care Act] emphasizes more on prevention/ disease [and] prevention/health promotion. [We should] prepare the nurses for this role." In addition, we should prepare nurses to care for the large numbers of aging baby boomers with "more bereavement training to help with what's coming over the next 30 years" and more education "about end-stage illness and end of life."

Nurses continue to feel that students lack critical-thinking skills and that "problem-solving exercises" might better prepare them. Finally, students should learn more about "universal precautions: Hair off the uniform, no nails, clean clothes...etc."

Many expressed that classes should "incorporate leadership opportunities" and "professional development." They stressed the importance of "prepar[ing] students on the needed education for mobility upward in the nursing field" and "integrat[ing] leadership activities/ expectations early in the program."

Reading these comments (and many similar ones from the survey), I got a sense that schools are educating students in very different ways. I was surprised to learn that not every student is provided with the same general background. I don't advocate a standardized, rote curriculum across the country. However, we all should emphasize basic components of nursing such as preventive care, leadership, and gerontology. Perhaps we could benefit from slightly more standardization across schools.

More Clinical

The need for more reality-based clinical experiences, more time in clinical practice, and practice in settings in addition to the hospital was echoed numerous times in the survey responses. Nurses clearly feel very strongly about the need to improve clinical experiences for students. One nurse responded, "Increase clinical hours. Don't expect to pump out high-quality nurses with little hours." The way clinical experiences are shaped for students is as important, if not more important, to nurse respondents as the number of hours students spend in clinical. One nurse observed, "Instructors should focus on questioning students on what they will be doing, then allow them to prepare and perform independently, only jumping in if necessary. Don't give excessive help as it hinders critical thinking."

Upon graduation, new nurses are not prepared to care for several patients because they only provide care for one or two patients while in school. One nurse suggested, "Have nursing students take a full patient load (overload)." In this way, students can learn "more of what it is like in reality. I feel new nurses are quickly becoming dismayed and overwhelmed because they weren't prepared for how hard the job is and the pressures involved." Another nurse added, "Each semester should emphasize the need for both time management and compassion for patients." Board exams should better reflect current practice. "Pressure the NCSBN/ NCLEX organizations to contemporize their testing plan/test to better reflect what is real."

Students need more practice communicating with families and patients. One nurse suggested, "Increase students' interactions with their patients, stay in the room with them as much as possible." It is also important, given changes in healthcare, that students receive "more comprehensive education regarding nursing practice in various settings— not only acute care."

One nurse wrote, "Since there is a shift to adult health and gerontology due to the aging population, home health nursing needs to be the bulk of nursing education." Another added, "Nurse practitioners must be authorized to oversee a home health plan of care."

Back to Basics

Interestingly, nurse respondents placed some emphasis on the need for learning skills and returning to the basics of nursing care without sacrificing the advances we have made in providing cutting-edge care and using technology. Some believe we should "enforce basic nursing skills" and "focus on students achieving a certain set of skills in order to finish rather than just a specific number of hours to ensure experience is obtained." Another nurse said, "Ensure that every student nurse is proficient in all basic nursing functions such as urinary catheter insertion, IV [intravenous] insertion, all types of medication administration."

While I agree that we must return to the basics and emphasize their importance to students, I don't agree that students must be proficient in all nursing skills prior to graduation. I think the emphasis should be on critical thinking and decision-making. Many skills, if need be, can be learned on the job depending on the work the nurse chooses to do.

Reevaluate the DNP

Nurses have very strong opinions about the doctorate of nursing practice, either strongly in favor ("[We] need to see how the new BSN-to-DNP clinicians do! I hope I am pleasantly surprised.") or strongly against ("Quit jamming the DNP down the throats of NPs."). Some feel we should "continue to have [the] master's degree as entry level for NPs."

Many expressed that it is unfair and ill advised to require the DNP to practice as an advanced practice registered nurse (APRN). One nurse wrote:

> [I] recommend that nurses be required to have 3 to 5 years experience as an RN before going on to an advanced degree. They need to know the basics and learn the art of critical thinking and communication and collaboration before being on their own as an NP.

Many are skeptical about whether the DNP will make a difference in patient care. Some feel that programs that allow students to obtain graduate degrees before having sufficient time practicing as RNs do not prepare nurses to practice effectively. As observed by one nurse:

> Do not push so hard for doctoral degrees as it makes us look like we want to be MDs but couldn't for some reason, or we look jealous. I believe patients are already confused with the number of doctors that are not medical docs.

Rethink Accelerated, For-Profit, and Online Programs

Special programs that accelerate students becoming nurses or bypass traditional classroom experiences were not generally viewed favorably by nurse respondents. Online programs ("Eliminate the online education") and for-profit programs ("Eliminate for-profit schools from basic nursing education") were not considered effective in providing a comprehensive nursing education. On a different note, one nurse observed that "online education should be more affordable at all levels. I could not complete a doctorate even online due to cost."

On a graduate level, many see a need for nurses to obtain experience before pursuing advanced degrees, particularly in advanced practice programs. "Stop the accelerated programs for non-nurses to get an advanced degree. For the most part, these nurses are not prepared to function in the role of NP if they have not been a nurse first." Another added, "Stop promoting RN-NP programs since even the experienced RN has difficulty adjusting to [the] NP role."

Interprofessional Education

Nurses seem to recognize the value of interprofessional education ("Have medical and nursing students together for similar courses"), even to the point of enlisting the assistance of non-nurses to educate nurses ("Include non-nursing healthcare professionals in education of nurses, [such as] physicians, psychologists, physical therapists"). This is another example of how nurse respondents feel students could receive better preparation for the real world they will encounter after graduation. Retired nurses can "talk about the hints and tricks of the trade as well as the 'art' of nursing."

"More interprofessional education (e.g., with medical, pharmacy, dietician, physical therapy, etc.)" can help students learn "problem-solving techniques for interpersonal conflict both intraprofessionally and inter-professionally" and teach them "conflict management, leadership training, and professionalism." Certainly, nursing students should be educated alongside students from other disciplines, when appropriate. However, let's be careful when we consider having faculty outside of nursing teach our students. There is always a place for that, but nursing faculty should supervise the content. Interestingly, in the early days, physicians taught our students, and that did not serve us well in terms of the physician-nurse relationship or of elevating the profession.

Make Education Affordable

Nurses report that continuing one's education can be very costly and recommend that more scholarships and tuition-reimbursement programs be made available. "[We] need to make advanced degrees more financially attainable. If the salary increase won't make it worthwhile, we don't pursue advanced education." One nurse suggested, "Create more scholarship opportunities for those seeking to attend higher priced continuing education programs." A few contend that ladders, such as those we have begun to provide for diploma and associate degree nurses to obtain the BSN degree, should be provided for nurses "from BSN to PhD with dissertation funding and nursing educator grants to move the best and the brightest quickly into practice." However, most responded that ladders move students through too quickly without providing sufficient experience working as nurses first.

Many suggest combining resources to provide better career counseling for new graduates and encouraging them to explore nursing opportunities outside of the hospital. We should reconsider the traditional view that everyone needs 1 year in medical-surgical nursing before they can seriously work as nurse.

Assist With Employment

Nurses request more assistance in career planning and to find jobs. Nurses responded, "Nursing education should link their resources and connections to help graduates find employment after graduation" and "add classes in career planning, interviewing, and résumé writing." We may not be as transparent as we think we are about the job market. One nurse urged educators to "be honest about how hard it will be to get that first job. Make everyone work as a CNA [certified nurse' s aide] in a hospital setting so they can get experience!"

I'm not sure I agree that students must work as nurse's aides or in some other medical capacity prior to or during nursing school. The mind-set with which someone performs those jobs is very different from that of a professional nurse. Frequently, nurse educators must work hard to dispel preconceived ideas before professional nursing concepts can take hold. However, many hospitals in particular want new nurses to come with experience, so work as a CNA or in another para-nursing capacity might help prepare new or prospective nurses for the hospital environment and to obtain jobs.

Pay Nurse Educators

The issue of pay was predominant among nurses who responded to the survey. "Academia needs to raise the salaries of teachers to attract more nurses who are good teachers." Many respondents expressed that if nurse educators received better pay, schools could attract better qualified educators. "Increase the pay!" wrote one. "Acknowledge the importance of pay and the relationship to being able to recruit more faculty and subsequently educate more nurses!" This applies to full-time as well as adjunct faculty. Clinical faculty, especially, should be paid and treated fairly so that the most expert nurses teach students in clinical settings. Said one respondent:

> Pay nurse educators what they are worth, including full-time faculty and adjuncts. Better pay may be more likely to attract nurses to nursing education. Currently, nurses can make more money working in many clinical settings than as educators and don't require advanced education in many cases.

Another nurse said, "Hire, involve, and pay adjunct faculty appropriately to enhance the integration of classroom knowledge and clinical experience. We can no longer teach students everything they need to know in the classroom." One nurse exhorted, "Continue to train RNs to be potential instructors, but set high expectations and screening. (Don't just accept a warm body to keep a program afloat.)"

Prepare Faculty to Teach

There is a general sense that not all faculty are well-prepared to teach and should take education courses and maintain clinical currency. Yes, schools should "hire academics who are clinical providers or have their hands in the real world." But they should "better educate the nurses who teach. They might need to take education courses."

In addition, nurse respondents thought that nurse educators should be active clinically "in some capacity to teach others the real world" and "ensure that classroom and clinical faculty are expert clinicians in the subject matter of the course and able to assist students in thinking critically about their patients." New faculty and new clinical adjuncts should be offered "an education forum…or be provide[d] [with] an adequate orientation."

Increase Rigor

There is concern about rigor, in general. Students are not required to "move beyond minimum competencies." We owe it to ourselves and our patients to enact "more stringent evaluation of students [and] fail them when appropriate" and "more strenuous certification preparation."

We do not use sufficient scrutiny when evaluating students for admission. ("Require an aptitude test prior to being accepted into a nursing program," one nurse suggested.) Then, we graduate them before they are ready to accept the responsibilities of the professional nurse. (One nurse exhorted, "Stop graduating nurses who do not believe that they are accountable for patient outcomes.") In sum, many nurses feel we should "establish and enforce high standards for and within all nursing programs."

Nurses are being moved through nursing programs too expediently, with a loss of educational rigor. One respondent noted, "Stop graduating students who cannot write a sentence [or] paragraph. Medical records matter!" Students are also encouraged to pursue graduate work too quickly. One nurse said there should be a "minimum of 3 years experience before allowance in ARNP programs."

Requiring "stepwise national boards throughout nursing education programs" and more rigorous licensing ("Licensing should move back to the more difficult but comprehensive exam to ensure the competency of new grads.") might serve to weed out people who are not suited to or capable of becoming nurses. "If people wash out, then they have not spent quite so much money before discovering that nursing is not for them."

One nurse suggested, "Focus on why to become and why *not* to become a nurse before going to school. Screen out those not appropriate."

Practice

Nurse respondents proposed solutions to several practice issues that remain with us despite the years of recognition and attempts to resolve or eliminate them.

Improve Professionalism and Image

Nurse respondents offer a variety of solutions to the problems encountered in clinical practice beyond the nursing school. There is a great deal of concern about the image nurses portray to the public, to each other, and to other professionals. The issue of professionalism transcends nursing education and overlaps into practice. If students are admitted to schools of nursing without regard for their character or ability and are assisted to move through programs to graduate, then practice settings are left to cope with incompetent nurses who impair our image.

Nurse respondents propose remedying this by "conduct[ing] thorough screenings of character, performance/references, and periodic drug screenings during educational programs" and "establish[ing] dress-code policies for street-clothes settings, about tightness of clothing, cleavage exposed, socks with shoes, etc."

While many schools do enforce a dress code, some nurses think we should "[have] national minimal expectations of appearance/uniform to promote a more positive nursing identity and image." It is our duty to "teach nurses to respect the profession—including how they portray themselves in their personal and public lives." To do this, experienced nurses should "be good role model[s], i.e., lose weight, exercise, stop smoking, etc." and "[demonstrate] professional etiquette."

If we "discipline those who are unprofessional," "[refuse to] tolerate any negative talk about difficult patients," and "start with the basics: lowering voices in the clinical setting, focusing on patient care instead of another nurse's love-life, and not wearing fake nails or nail polish," then perhaps we can convince the public of our professional status.

Some nurses think that to "regain [our] identity, [we must return to a] uniform for nurses and restrict nonclinical departments from wearing scrubs." One nurse wrote:

> The image of nursing is suffering via [the] lack of being readily identifiable, [the] general public's confusion [regarding] who is a nurse, the various levels of nursing, [the] decline in professional appearance, [and] increased tolerance of visible tattoos, nose rings and other body piercings, foul language, etc.

One nurse commented, "Students should be required to sit in on board hearings of nurses accused of violations or attend required symposiums." Presumably, doing so would help students avoid making similar mistakes in the future.

Increase Self-Care and Reduce Burnout

Survey respondents believed we should support and nurture new nurses and promote their involvement in the profession by encouraging them to join our organizations and actively participate. We should "encourage self-care to avoid burnout and attrition from the profession." Once again, the notion that we eat our young comes to the forefront. If so many nurses decry this behavior, then why is it still happening? Nurse respondents exhort us to "care for each other" and "support and work together."

Nurses should "create an attitude where it focuses importance on taking care of oneself. Remember to take meal and toilet breaks so that nurses don't make themselves martyrs." It is important to our survival as a profession that we "care for new and old nurses with support and understanding" and "promote collegiality and collaboration among nurses at all levels" and "intraprofessional collaboration."

One nurse explained:

> Working as a nurse can be very stressful, and as a result, nurses are sometimes burned out and suffer many health problems. In addition, becoming a nurse is not an easy process and many nurses face a hostile environment once in the workplace. I have felt threatened personally for reporting alleged abuse of residents. Nurses are oftentimes treated with an iron hand and are disciplined

more frequently than other members of the nursing staff. [Sometimes] ancillary workers have more rights than nurses and are treated more fairly.

Bullying and incivility appear to be alive and well in the workplace, and nurses seem to be suffering as a result. Nurses must "demonstrate courage to confront and deal with lateral violence. NO BULLYING, period." It is important that we educate ourselves about preventing bullying and hold "group sessions to address the work-life balance and bullying." Furthermore, "We need more regulations regarding bullying in the nurse practice act, not just the ANA Ethics Code."

Nurse respondents feel strongly that there should be "zero tolerance for bullying [and that healthcare agencies should] conduct a root-cause analysis of bullying allegations." One nurse concluded that "nurses as a whole need education about mentoring and encouragement to stop 'eating their young' and bullying."

Pay Nurses What They're Worth

Not only do nurse educators need to receive better pay, but practicing nurses should be more fairly compensated for their work and receive monetary incentives. In addition, we should return to "salary differentials for BSN versus ADN to reward ongoing education," and should improve nurse work hours.

Some nurses expressed that we are not sufficiently "compensated for wellness work outside of hospitals" and don't adequately "reimburse for community RNs to follow up discharged patients." Another added, "[There needs to be] advance billing for nursing services. Otherwise we will never have true power if we can't demonstrate capital value."

Nurses appear to be unhappy with unionization in academe ("Work to remove unionization for nursing faculty, remove [the] tenure option for clinical instructors and pay them well.") and in practice ("Stop being in unions."). Nurses need "incentives...to stay in their current positions" and "more money with chances to make more." Another added, "Hospitals need to develop meaningful clinical ladders with rewards (monetary and recognition) for nurses working at the bedside."

Enhance Collaboration and Communication

Nurse respondents commented on what new graduates should know when starting to practice. In their view, nurses should emerge from school knowing how to work collaboratively and comfortably with other disciplines, including ancillary staff, within their healthcare setting. They should have excellent oral and written communication skills and be skilled in conflict management and resolution.

Nurses should be knowledgeable regarding what other staff bring to patient care and how to best utilize them. "New graduates should know more about RNs, APRNs, PAs, and MDs—their similarities and differences," noted one respondent. Conversely, "Physicians need to be educated on the RN's role and how much liability we have in our patients' care," "be encouraged to use RN visual evaluations to help keep chronic patients out of clinics and ERs," and "take each concern seriously and listen when a concern is voiced by an RN." In general, we "[need] more teamwork between MDs and RNs" along with "interdisciplinary projects" and "more peer and interdisciplinary communication skills training." Nurses—especially those who have not had the benefit of education in an interprofessional environment—should be trained "to interact with physicians and interdisciplinary professionals."

Increased collaboration and communication doesn't apply only to interactions with other healthcare disciplines, but with each other. "Connect nurse researchers with practicing nurses and provide time for them to collaborate," suggested one respondent. It is important to have "education and awareness of modesty, respect, and collaboration—and that starts from the top with educators, regulating bodies, [and] nurse organizations." One nurse stated that we should "allow bedside nurses paid time outside of bedside nursing to have some administrative duties [because] there is always a lack of understanding between bedside nursing and nursing administration."

"Allow[ing] interdepartmental cross-pollination, walking in [an] other's shoes to experience nursing profession from all aspects," can help "create workplace groups [in which] all medical professionals [work] cooperatively [to] problem solve patient and workplace issues." Mixing "the generations of nursing" can help to pass on the nursing traditions worth saving and the wisdom that comes with experience.

Reevaluate Use of Ancillary Staff

Although most nurses seem to value ancillary staff such as licensed practical nurses (LPN), certified nurse's aides (CNAs), medical assistants (MAs), and others, many believe that some functions of the RN are inappropriately being taken over by ancillary staff. The former support the "need to hire more CNAs so RNs can have time to plan the care of the patient rather than do CNA work constantly." The latter contend that we should "hire more nurses and less CNAs" and "clarify to the nurse's aides that they are just that and not fully fledged nurses." In addition, there is a need to "re-address the role and need for LPNs in many sectors."

One nurse was adamant:

> Way too many registered nurses are being replaced by MAs and it is having a very detrimental effect on the health outcomes of our population. We must continue to advocate for the registered nurses in our healthcare settings and support their continuing involvement in all aspects of our healthcare and our healthcare settings so our voice continues to be heard. We are the best advocates our patients have, and if we give up that role, it is a definite detriment to our patients.

Redistribute and Reduce Workload

Nurse workload continues to be a problem for nurses practicing clinically. To aid in this, nurses suggested we "go back to 8-hour shifts for safety and also to help prevent nurse burnout" and "quit forcing people into 12-hour shifts. Folks are exhausted, mean, and cranky."

The high ratio of patients to one nurse remains staggering given the high technology and acuity needs of patients today. "The work environment has to be conducive to eliminate cutting corners," noted one respondent. The nurse-patient ratio is a problem in many settings. One responded suggested "Implement[ing] policy to decrease [the] patient-nurse ratio throughout the healthcare arena [including] nursing home, hospital, and specialty units." One nurse went further: "Set patient ratio on a federal level and [do] not allow hospital administration to deviate from the guidelines."

Nurses need to be supported to prevent them from leaving due to burnout. Nurses suggested that employers "[provide] resources for nurses who are burned out to help them adapt without losing them" and "provide more scheduling flexibility to reduce attrition and burnout." Another said, "Administrators should strive to provide flexibility in work/shift scheduling" and "rethink the current workflow design." This nurse continued:

> Primary nursing is not working with 12-hour days, 3 days per week, because the nurse usually does not work 2 days together. Primary nursing may work with 8 hours and a 5-day workweek, but let's consider other formats. Maybe team nursing can be resurrected. I know it worked well when I was on the medical-surgical units.

Another suggested the following:

> Standardize[d] patient load for nurses depend[ing] upon the care needed for the patient. Maybe using a point system for patients and the care they need. Then a nurse's caseload would be dependent upon the maximum number of points one can safely handle. This would make more difficult or needy patients have more points and less needy patients, less points.

Promote Lifelong Learning

We promote continuing education (CE) and lifelong learning among our students, but respondents say we don't make it mandatory after graduation. They advocate the following:

- **Requiring continuing education units in every state:**

  "Encourage ALL states to mandate continuing education for nurses."

  "Change mandatory CEs frequently."

- **Providing incentives to healthcare agencies for giving tuition reimbursement:**

  "Educate in school and continue once in practice."

- **Giving working staff the time and opportunity to engage in professional growth activities:**

  "Ensure that nursing students, educators, and nursing staff are exposed to the latest technology and develop competency in using technology."

Nurse respondents wrote in strong terms about "encourag[ing] scholarship at [the] bedside," "hav[ing] educational sessions on new changes in practice," and "focus[ing] on how the staff nurse can expand his/her role after [the] 'task mastery' phase. Encourage them to expand their roles at the bedside in order to reduce turnover." To do so, organizations could "support enough staffing so current staff can go to conferences, etc. We are frequently denied time off." Organizations could also "[provide] incentives for research."

There should be "incentives/awards for facilities to be flexible with schedules for those employees going back to school." In addition, "workplaces could offer incentive pay or raises for higher degrees." One nurse commented, "Recruit facilities and individuals to provide scholarships for working mothers to further education."

Promote Leadership

Nurses were vehement with regard to issues around nursing leadership. They expressed that nurses should be encouraged to become leaders and involved in the profession. We should "support and encourage leadership and research" and "provide more support for mid- and upper-level leaders to take risks to lead improvement projects" and "develop both practice expertise and leadership skills."

One nurse exhorted that we "make engagement and evidenced-based practice a priority [and] define leadership by actions and attributes, not position and power." Others commented that all nurses should "be open to change and innovative methods and solutions" and learn "how to work with committees" to "think outside the box."

Several discussed evidence-based practice (EBP). Many urged the implementation of systems to ensure that nurses based practice on EBP and knew how to enact change. One nurse suggested, "Require a written proposal for initiating system-wide change to an evidence-based practice," and another asserted, "promote assertiveness and promote competency of nurses."

Nurses felt that bad leaders should be held "accountable…[they] are the most destructive force in healthcare." Good leaders "lead by example," "encourage individualism and thought," and "become more involved, go to the front lines and see what is happening." One nurse recommended "an independent institutional leadership for nursing." That might help "nursing leaders [have] a more realistic view of nursing today." Another said:

> The nurse leaders of the past were too focused in what type of degree one should have rather than expanding the role of the nurse in society. This has hurt nursing and women in this profession. [We] need more visionary leadership.

Another nurse suggested that we "remove executives that do not have a nursing background." Still another recommended we

> form healthcare communities in which patients have access to nurses as the gatekeepers, triaging them to the appropriate professionals as necessary (physicians, physical therapists, etc.).

Nurses think their colleagues should "speak out in their clinical settings to impact administration's decisions to save resources" and "push for increased nursing decision-making." Others said that "we need to propose and get funding for more demonstration projects with real research to measure outcomes" and "develop a truly nursing vision of healthcare restructuring" while we "continue to push for change."

Several nurses wrote that there should be "peer reviews of administrative supervisors and leadership," that we should "listen to those who do the job—the bedside nurses," and generally ensure that the voice of the direct care nurse is heard. One nurse recommended "develop[ing] the professional organizations to reflect the needs of staff nurses, not educators and administrators, including mandating that over 50% of any organizational board is composed of staff nurses."

Policy

Nurse respondents were adamant that it is incumbent upon all nurses to get involved in nursing and health policy decision-making. They advocated that we instill students with the importance and wherewithal to fully participate in policy activities.

Educate Students and Nurses

Nurse respondents had many suggestions for engaging both students and nurses in policy making. Here are just a few:

- "[Direct] more continuing education on health policy toward currently practicing nurses."
- "Expect civic engagement."
- "[Offer] a political action class."

Respondents also believed we should help students understand that "nursing is a political force for change" and should provide "earlier and consistent exposure…to [the] basics of health policy and personal professional advocacy so nurses are not so resistant to grassroots communication with their elected officials."

Nurses should be prepared "to serve on boards and commissions" and become "educated on current issues in healthcare policy, and how each nurse, regardless of the level, is impacted by laws." Respondents recommended we "teach students to advocate not only for the patient but for themselves as a profession" and "encourage students to be risk takers/advocates/leaders within healthcare and healthcare policy" by "[instituting a] mandatory curriculum on politics, lobbying, legislative issues, etc." and "provid[ing] information about healthcare policy and issues."

Become Politically Active

Nurses think it is necessary for "policy makers...to understand that increasing [the] length of education required for NPs will reduce participation and access." We must "organize bedside nurses as a political force for change—staffing, patient safety, social justice" and "provide more support to nurses who want to be politically active [and] more money so nurses can return to school and further their education."

Nurses recommend more discussion and emphasis "[on] political action at the hospital level," "on health policy in nursing education at all levels," and "from schools and employers regarding policy issues and professional membership."

Work With Nursing Organizations

One nurse proposed that "regulation within the practice has gotten too top heavy and cumbersome [with] too many questionable political ties. Organizations that support nurses should have more weight and [be] given more governing power of the profession."

This seems contradictory to the pervasive view among nurse respondents that the leaders of nursing organizations don't always know what is happening at the bedside and that they have too much governing power over the profession. If this respondent intended this statement to mean that nursing organizations should have the governing power over the profession *as opposed to* politicians who make decisions that affect us, then I heartily agree.

Many believe the profession should "support autonomy" and "promote [nurse] involvement in state-level professional practice issues" by "campaign[ing] to get nurses involved and joining organizations."

Lobby and Discuss Legislation

Nurses wrote thoughtfully of the need to "lobby our legislators and the public" and "discuss laws and legislations that impact healthcare proactively." They propose that nurses serve on advisory councils and legislative committees, engaging in "more legislative action from nurses at [the] state level and national level (making a positive difference)."

Furthermore, "We need to put more nurses in state legislatures and congressional seats." Employers should support these efforts by "allow[ing] RNs time to testify [and] lobby for best practice for health policy" and "increasing funding for nursing (not union) agenda lobbying efforts."

According to the nurse respondents, we should lobby for the following:

- "Equality of reimbursement for advanced practice nurses"

- "Removal of practice restrictions"

- "More representation on the federal committees that deal with direct healthcare policy making"

- "Socialized medicine without the middlemen insurance companies"

- "Reasonable limits on [the] number of patients nurses can care for at one time in different types of settings"

- "An expanded role that allows us to practice to the fullest extent of our education"

One nurse spoke for many when suggesting that we must unify if our efforts are to be effectual: "We must promote mandatory membership to a unified lobbying voice at a national level, then strongly encourage state-level membership. Dual membership should be granted to new graduates for reasonable fees." Another added, "We must unify our voice and stop separating our lobbying and accrediting bodies."

Promote Change

However we choose to do it, nurses are expected to "promote legislature change" and "whistleblower legislation." Further, we should "create a legal defense fund so nurse whistleblowers have recourse to expose the problems at their hospitals." We should also "use any available political clout to change the staggering pay disparity for home care and community clinic nurses."

Understand Reimbursement Practices

Nurses think it is time that we all had a better understanding of how reimbursement affects care, the various sources of reimbursement, and how they work. Specifically, nurse respondents cited the need to "understand payment of Medicare," "understand payer sources," and "teach nurses how to bill the insurance."

Home health nurses have worked with reimbursement factors for many years. It is vital to know what will and will not be paid for when caring for patients in the home setting to avoid the occurrence or appearance of fraud or abuse of the Medicare system. Nurse practitioners and other APRNs certainly require knowledge of reimbursement practices to best serve their patients. One medication may cost far less than another in the same class. A diagnostic test is probably not needed if performing it won't change the treatment plan. It is not unreasonable for nurses, regardless of setting, to have a better understanding than they have needed in the past of who pays for what so we can continue to effectively advocate for our patients.

Another nurse wrote specifically about "care/services provided to the elderly. We must look at ways to avoid increasing rates for the elderly. Where will they get extra cash to support cost-of-living and medical increases?"

Vote and Get Involved

Getting involved, particularly by voting, was viewed by the surveyed nurses as fundamental to promoting change. "Nurses [should] vote themselves and encourage others to vote." We should "encourage [students] to vote as part of professionalism (more focus at entry-level nursing school)," but "all nurses should take more political action" and "becom[e] more politically active in general—it's not something I enjoy, but I have found I must do it to advocate." The profession should take steps to "develop strategies for nurses to become more involved in policy development" and "encourage nurses and government entities to involve nurses in healthcare policy decisions."

We must "establish a presence amongst legislators and constituents regarding [the] nurses' role in policy." In addition, we must:

> Find creative ways (call-in hours, blogs, webinars) to get everyday, boots-on-the-ground nurses involved—either locally or nationally—and spread this experience to more of us. [We should] provide regular, relatively easy ways for nurses to get involved with healthcare policy; that will get more of us paying attention and being involved and adding our voices to policy decisions.

Another nurse said, "Find many more advocates for RNs and APNs at [the] state and national level. Don't let doctors have all the big politicians in their corners." Another added, "Find nurses who have succeeded in political fields and been elected to office to serve as role models and mentors."

Most nurses who responded to the question of how we could do better with regard to policy clearly emphasized the need to "get involved in politics at any level (letter writing, information sessions, running for office) [and] groom and support a cadre of nursing leaders for policy making." One nurse was adamant that "nursing organizations should never support a particular politician, ever!" I have to admit that I agree with that statement. Organizations should support policy, not politicians. Another agreed: "Stick with the issues, legislation, and advancement of nurses in a bipartisan fashion, careful to never alienate its members."

Some think our organizations are not involved enough. One wrote, "Nursing professional organizations [should] become involved in health-care policy."

"Opportunities to serve in political leadership roles" and for "prestigious nursing internships...regarding policy" can help educate nurses and increase nurse visibility in political arenas. Getting involved also includes "talk[ing] to the politicians that decide our fate through laws/regulations" and "spotlight[ing] issues for policy makers."

It is important that new nurses be introduced to involvement in policy early in their careers. "Somehow we have to bring new nurses along with us. Or maybe after a nurse's first year, [he or she] might be more ready to hear policy positions and how [he or she] can help." According to one nurse, it's key that we do the following:

Actively participate in our community, our professional association, and our policy settings so we have a voice that is heard loudly and clearly. We are the most respected group of professionals and we must not let anyone else speak for us.

Get the Word Out

Another way to make sure nurses' voices are heard is to "continue to publish in [the] lay press [about the] outcomes of APRN care" and "build upon society's perception of nurses being honest by being more visible (advertising)." It is important that "the public see how involved nurses are with policy making." Visibility of nurse involvement can help "mobilize public pressure on politicians for desired outcomes." We need to "use multiple media to communicate information about policy" and "highlight those nurses who are advising—and who are current—elected and appointed officials." We also must "inform nurses regularly on policy issues." One nurse said:

> Get the word out to the nurse at the bedside regarding changes in health policy and how it affects patient care and how these changes can affect the nurse/patient ratio in the future. Make nursing a partner in the process to improve care delivery so that we can have good patient outcomes and (hopefully) increased reimbursement.

Unify

The theme of unification pervades education, practice, and policy. With regard to policy, one nurse said we "need to start grassroots efforts to organize nurses with a political voice" because "nurses are often quiet when it comes to policy and the laws that affect healthcare and our citizens." Particularly in light of the changes in healthcare, "nurses need to be in the forefront of preventive care policies," "be more vocal and get involved in all policy, [including] local, regional, national, and international," and "speak with one voice, be unified."

To unify, we must "stop fighting among ourselves." One nurse observed, "We have not come together as nurses to help each other, so maybe [we should have] some national task forces to work on solutions." Not only should we feel obligated to "join an organization and be active," but we must "respond [to] calls for action from our professional organizations." If we have "one agency to define the role of practice for nurses and ARNPs as a whole, [this will] eliminate the state-to-state guidelines."

There is too much fragmentation of nursing organizations to enable us to speak with one voice. "Harness our collective strength," said one nurse. Another nurse suggested "[getting] rid of the smaller professional organizations and groups and band[ing] together for one loud voice" with "more coordination among nursing groups/organizations to promote consistency in implementation strategies." It is important that specialty groups be included as well, with "more communication among nurses at all levels and in all specialties regarding needed initiatives."

In addition to standardizing education, we should standardize our professional organizations and "unify the nursing certification bodies; there should only be one. ANCC and AANP and their members must merge before we have leverage against AMA and other medical powers for lobbying/scope of practice arguments." Another nurse summed it up as follows:

> Nursing needs to become one, united group that advocates for the patient and for the nursing profession. There are so many nursing groups…[I'm] not sure how to do this, but we should find a way to come together so we all have one strong voice.

Improve Our Professional Image

Some nurses discussed the need to redefine ourselves or to make what we do clearer to the public. One nurse noted the following:

> Nursing care plans and nursing diagnosis have been the flagship concept in nursing. But nursing care plans are ignored. How do we solve that? Nurse educators must meet to brainstorm a new overarching paradigm that sets us apart in what we offer patients. A nursing diagnosis—for

example, "potential for dehydration related to decreased fluid intake"—is obvious, and the steps to remedy that are always addressed by the physician—i.e., take IV fluids. Why are we restating that? Do we not trust that we have educated nurses to understand why IV fluids are ordered? I would have to spend more time thinking through a specific solution, but a start would be for nursing to truly find what can be our flagship contribution that is valued enough by ourselves and our professional counterparts—MDs, DOs, PTs, [and] pharmacists. That [should be] the platform upon which our professional expertise rests.

One nurse said, "Define [the] role of ARNPs at a federal level to allow for equality in practice." Another wrote, "Stress ANA and ICN nursing definitions." The need to define nursing as it exists today and as we want to see it in the future is of great concern to surveyed nurses. One replied:

What exactly is nursing, anyway? We can't get money for it if we can't define it better. Why are CPT codes the only way to record what care was given to a patient that counts? The AMA doesn't know what we do.

We require "better public relations/telling our story so [the] public knows what we do and that it's worthwhile." However, "creat[ing] clarity for [the] public requires us to have clarity within ourselves." Many nurses proposed that we do a better job of educating boards of healthcare organizations as well as politicians and legislators about what we do. "Educate boards of hospitals about what nursing is and nursing does. Have nurses present this." Another nurse was more specific: "Let's teach [the] public that nurses are scientists of the human condition, not just carers." We should "be more visible in the media" and have "TV public service announcements that highlight nursing in the 50s and 60s versus today's nurses, who utilize increasing technology and care for much sicker patients." We should help "patients/clients [know who we are and what we do by providing them] with lists of professionals and paraprofessionals that they may encounter" so that "consumers…know the value of nursing."

Promote Citizenship

Several survey respondents commented that nurses should be good citizens. They should, one nurse explained, "promote civic engagement and create an expectation of being a good nurse citizen—involvement in professional organizations, nursing policy, volunteer activities." Being a good nurse is not enough. Nurses must "be involved in community healthcare as a citizen, not just as a nurse."

Some nurses mentioned community and public health, in particular, as areas in which nurses could be good citizens. Respondents suggested "increas[ing] funding to nursing to bring back community and public health focus" and "promot[ing]...preventative healthcare via community nursing." Others urged nurses to "step up and design a role in national disasters and community disasters—Katrina, school shootings, etc."

Support APRNs

Several respondents wrote specifically about APRNs and their role in policy. Said one nurse, "advanced practice nurses...clinical nurse leaders [should be used] to their full abilities." One proposed that we "embrace advanced practice nursing as part of nursing by encourag[ing] more integration between national NP and national nursing organizations." Others said we should "continue to increase the use of advanced practice nurses in all settings while allowing them to practice with autonomy," "pass laws to allow APRNs to practice to their full potential," and "promote and demand independent practices for ARNPs in communities and within healthcare, permitting independent practice for APRNs."

Conclusion

It is plain that nurses have clear and substantial ideas regarding solutions to many of the issues that continue to confront the profession. Some of these ideas have already been translated into action. If we don't listen to the voices of nurses regarding the day-to-day issues we face individually and collectively, many of them may never be resolved.

PROPOSED SOLUTIONS

EDUCATION

Require BSN for entry to practice

Improve mentoring

Standardize nursing education

Emphasize theory and research

Broaden knowledge and incorporate liberal education concepts into discussions of nursing

Increase clinical time and patients per student

Ensure students learn and perform basics of nursing care

Reevaluate DNP

Rethink accelerated, online, and for-profit programs

Make education affordable

Assist with employment

Pay nurse educators what they are worth

Prepare faculty to teach

Require faculty practice

Increase rigor in admissions and academic expectations

NURSING PRACTICE

Improve professionalism and image

Increase self-care and reduce burnout

Pay nurses what they are worth

Enhance collaboration and communication inter- and intra-professionally

Reevaluate utilization of ancillary staff

Redistribute and reduce workload

Promote lifelong learning

Promote leadership

POLICY

Educate students and nurses about health policy

Become politically active

continues

Require nursing organizations to focus on policy, not politics

Get involved with nursing organizations

Lobby and discuss legislation

Promote change

Understand reimbursement practices

Vote and get involved

Get the word out

Unify

Improve professional image

Promote citizenship

Support APRNs

Reference

Institute of Medicine. (2010). *The future of nursing: Leading change, advancing health*. Washington, DC: The National Academies Press.

Chapter 7

Looking Toward the Future for Nursing Education

There were 30 girls, all second-year nursing students, going to Chess Hall, the nurses' dormitory, on the grounds of St. Stephen's Psychiatric Hospital. Most of them were not more than 20 years old and were from strict Jewish and Catholic families in Brooklyn, New York. Feeling "footloose" in rural Long Island in the winter of 1951 was a real treat for them. The professional staff was practicing the permissive psychology in vogue at the time, so nursing students would be largely unsupervised in the dormitories and during their leisure time.

After a 4-hour drive from the Brooklyn Central Hospital, the bus entered the long macadam driveway of St. Stephen's. It was dusk, and the white steeple of the six-story gray administration building came into view. Hawks circled the steeple. "Any minute, Boris Karloff will appear," Amy Taft said with a giggle. Sara Friedman was the first to alight from the bus. She was approached by a short Asian man in a tan sleeveless shirt. He stopped in front of a large elm tree about 100 feet away. "Which way to the nurses' residence, please sir?" she asked, and was startled to notice that he was talking to the tree. She quickly backed away, her new stadium boots crunching the dry, cold leaves surrounding the tree. The man did not respond or stop talking to the tree. Sara shivered and returned to the group, now outside the bus. Dropping her arms in submission, she sighed. "Oy vey," she said.

A woman in a lab coat and fashionable harlequin eyeglasses arrived and took charge of the students. And so a month of psych rotation began. The weekdays were spent in class. Lectures on medications and treatment of schizophrenia were given by the staff physicians. A class on how to comport oneself on the wards didn't receive much attention, although the handsome young psychiatric resident explaining the procedure did. Later, I sang with the radio while studying the anatomy and physiology of the brain, sitting at an old wobbly desk in the small, old-fashioned library of Chess Hall. My thoughts wandered back to the parting from my boyfriend at the train station. He was off to fight in Korea. "See you at graduation, I hope," he had said as he shifted the heavy canvas duffel bag to his right shoulder and boarded the train.

Many of the themes related to education that were prevalent from 1900 to 2000 resound today. Nurses remain concerned that students are not learning to think critically, are not grounded in a broad liberal education (at least not enough to purport themselves as professionals), and do not get sufficient clinical preparation to face the realities once they graduate. Nurses still seek standardization of nursing education and full-time and clinical faculty who are current in nursing and prepared to teach. There is a lack of attention by nursing students to research, theory, policy, and the basics of nursing care. Many respondents continue to believe that we should spend more time educating students about nursing specialties and increase the emphasis on community care.

The fragmentation of programs and the options for graduate education and continuing education are still part of the conversation. In addition, the lack of rigor in whom we admit and retain among nursing students is at issue. The cost of education, remuneration for faculty, and interprofessional education may seem like newer issues, but they are essentially old issues reframed for a modern audience. Incivility is a big problem, but we have made room for more men and minorities in nursing education—although not nearly as much as one would think, given the age of the profession and modern social mores. We've also gone to great lengths to make veterans welcome in our schools; a positive change.

Critical Thinking

We frequently throw the words "critical thinking" around in schools and colleges of nursing. They have become a sort of mantra for what separates students learning to be registered nurses from ancillary personnel. The RN is supposed to critically assess the patient, develop the plan of care, and coordinate all the necessary elements to deliver the care and evaluate its effectiveness. Nurse educators work hard to find and use methodologies to assess whether students have learned to think critically and whether they have grown and developed in this area between starting nursing classes and graduating.

I don't think we have been able to measure critical thinking successfully. As they say, "the proof is in the pudding." I don't know that we can measure whether a student has improved in this area until that student is actually caring for patients on his or her own, in charge of what happens. Case analysis, however, can help students learn to problem-solve and apply theory to real-world scenarios. Simulation experiences and clinical practica can give us an inkling of critical thinking, but until nurses are legally responsible for the care they provide, I don't think we can have a true picture of how well they can make critical decisions.

Rigor

Part of the problem has to do with rigor—rigor in how and whom we admit and rigor regarding how we evaluate students and allow or not allow them to progress while in school. Nurse leaders agonized about rigor during the early days of the profession, as evidenced in Chapter 1, "Nurses Are Made Not Born: Educational Reform Frames the Profession (1900–1935), Chapter 2, "Rising from the Depths: We Are Not Subservient (1935–1970)," and Chapter 3, "Clinicians, Scientists, and Scholars: Separate but Equal (1970–2000)." There was controversy about whether programs were too structured and too rigorous, preventing students from thinking creatively or making their own decisions. As a profession, we seem to constantly bounce back and forth about how much is too much or too little rigor.

Many survey respondents agreed that we admit students who have neither the academic ability nor the character to be effective and safe nurses and that, once these students are admitted, we do too much hand-holding and spoon-feeding. I recently participated on a committee of administrators of schools of nursing who debated whether we should report the NCLEX board scores for second-time test-takers bundled with scores from first-time test-takers. The argument in favor was that the first-time test score was not an adequate reflection on the school. The reasoning was many first-time test-takers fail because they do not take the test seriously, but once they fail, they begin to study for the exam. The schools arguing in favor felt that it is a poor and inaccurate reflection on them if they have a high first-time test-taker failure rate. Those who spoke against combining the scores argued that not only would this give a skewed picture to the public of which schools graduated competent nurses, but that the second-time pass rate would more likely reflect the student's study skills than the rigor of the academic program.

We seem eager to accept anyone who will pay in both for-profit and not-for-profit programs. We offer programs online, in hybrid format, with accelerated options, and using any innovation we can devise to make nursing education as convenient as possible for potential students. I don't disagree that we should try to accommodate our students. And realistically, schools have to obtain tuition dollars to stay in business. However, I do think that we may be sacrificing rigor in some cases. We can still offer innovative and convenient programs that enforce high standards. So many people apply to nursing programs throughout the country every year. We turn potential students away. Can we not afford, then, to accept only the best and the brightest? Perhaps if we did so, we would be able to observe critical thinking taking place in the very first nursing class.

What is so wrong about telling students who are clearly not suited to nursing that perhaps they should rethink their choice? Many other countries require qualifying examinations, and students who don't meet the required score cannot enter a particular field of study. I am not suggesting that someone who wants to be a nurse should not have the opportunity to apply for a nursing program. I have seen a few students throughout the years who did not have strong academic backgrounds but managed to excel in nursing school. However, I think we do students, faculty, the profession, and most importantly, patients, a great disservice when we bend over backward to admit and retain students who are clearly unfit to be nurses. (By unfit, I mean academically incapable.)

Broad Liberal Education

Early nurse leaders felt strongly that nursing students should be given a broad liberal education, including the arts and humanities as well as the sciences. Nursing students should have a thirst for knowledge and want to become what we now call "lifelong learners." It was thought that students should know English literature and be prepared to speak and write well. There was a concern even in the early 1900s that students could not speak and write well, despite being native English speakers.

Today, while students in associate degree and baccalaureate nursing programs are required to have a liberal arts background and to take biology, anatomy and physiology, microbiology, and often chemistry and other sciences, we do not tend to require them to use what they've learned in the arts and humanities once they begin nursing classes. Moreover, we often neglect to inject rigor into their oral and written skills in favor of their clinical skills. Some faculty argue that nurses don't need to write in complete sentences due to the advent of the electronic health record (EHR). If we are merely preparing nurses to perform tasks and chart in the EHR, then why do they need to learn how to think critically and why should they be awarded baccalaureate degrees? It is embarrassing to the profession for nurses to have poor grammar and to be uncomfortable talking to other professionals. I think the lack of emphasis on writing, speaking articulately, and reading literature both from within and outside the profession is highly contributory to the image the public has of nurses.

Many nurses believe that we do not put enough emphasis on research, theory, or health policy in undergraduate education. I am a great proponent of evidence-based practice. However, since we began to emphasize it in nursing undergraduate curricula, research—how it's conducted, how to critically analyze it, and how knowing about it contributes to our professional image—seems to have been pushed out, sometimes to the point where it his hardly mentioned. Undergraduates don't need to conduct research studies, but they do need to know how to use research to support the work they do. They also should know how to read journal articles from within and outside of nursing and be able to separate the wheat from the chaff. To do so, they must understand what real and rigorous research is. Which research-based conclusions are worth paying attention to and incorporating into one's practice?

There remains controversy regarding whether nursing students should learn nursing and other theories. Personally, I don't understand why this is even a question. Every profession has theoretical underpinnings. If we don't learn the theories supporting what we do, how can we call ourselves professionals? We might as well be technicians. Understanding theories outside the discipline helps us to see that nursing does not operate in a vacuum. We require knowledge of psychology, sociology, language, history, etc., to be able to interpret what we encounter in day-to-day practice. How can we say we practice holistically when we don't understand anything beyond nursing?

Nurse respondents were very mixed with regard to the value of learning about nursing theories. They either love them or hate them. Im and Chang (2012) state:

> Although the priority of nursing science tends to be weighted to research these days, the coexistence of these three components [theory, research, and practice] is essential for advances in nursing science. We need to continue our efforts to link research and practice to theories and to work on the specifics that could be easily translated into our research and practice (p. 161)...Grand theories will play an important role in defining our discipline; middle-range theories will play an essential role in nursing research; and situation-specific theories will play an imperative role in nursing research and practice with diverse populations and situations, especially for those who are underserved in current health care systems. (p. 162)

Now more than ever, it is important for nursing students to have at least a basic understanding of health policy. In past years, knowledge of this seemed to be a divider between nurse leaders and others. The nurse leaders had made a point of learning about health policy and how nursing fit into it or was affected by it. This is still somewhat true. However, nurses on the front lines of care must understand the implications of the ACA. In addition, most need to know about Medicare and other insurance and how they affect the patient's ability to follow the plan of care—obtain their medicines, follow up with providers, etc. Policy remains a topic mostly geared to the graduate level, with some information integrated throughout the curriculum.

In addition to these areas, undergraduate nurses need a working knowledge of business, finance, economics, and organizational structure and behavior. While doing research for my previous book (Neal-Boylan, 2013), I found that new nurses often had more or at least as much trouble understanding the organization for which they worked than they did nursing care. We cannot make the undergraduate curriculum go on for years and years, but we do need to reevaluate how we currently use our class time and review where our emphases are and whether they should be updated to meet current needs.

Community Nursing Care

Changes in society and in healthcare are going to require changes in nursing. Although the majority of patient care has taken place in the community for a long time, nursing education has often viewed community and home health classes as stepchildren, sometimes integrating concepts or using acute care studies adapted to discuss community care. For years, economic changes have driven shortened hospital stays and increased skilled care provided in the home. However, nursing students rarely get enough exposure to home healthcare, nor are we good at instilling appreciation for what home care nurses do or encouraging new graduates to pursue home care. With increasing emphasis on prevention, public health—which in the early years was a focal point in nursing—is likely to have more priority. Epidemiology as well as the unique aspects of delivering care in the home and community should regain center stage in nursing education programs for undergraduates.

To properly educate nursing students about community health, it is necessary to have faculty with this experience. Having worked in home health for many years, I know that it is not just hospital care transplanted in the home (Neal-Boylan, 2008), nor is it simply taking vital signs and filling medication boxes. Home and community health nursing practices are unique unto themselves, and nurses going into those fields must feel confident in their skills and be comfortable making autonomous decisions. I still believe that new graduates need a good year of precepted time in the home setting because so much of the practice relies on the nurse's independent assessment and judgment. However, if community health nursing courses within schools of nursing are revamped to truly reflect the skills needed to practice competently in the home, then perhaps a long preceptorship will be less necessary.

We are hopeful that before long, APRNs will be able to sign plans of care and certify Medicare patients to receive home healthcare. The Home Health Care Planning Improvement Act ("Policy brief," 2014) is an effort toward accomplishing this. This is another good reason nurses in their basic nursing education programs should gain a detailed understanding of how reimbursement works and how orders are given and received.

Nursing Specialties

With the advent of the Affordable Care Act, nurse educators are beginning to appreciate the importance of ensuring that nursing students are prepared to practice in the community. In addition, new graduates are having difficulty finding hospital jobs immediately upon graduation. Many reluctantly migrate to work in other areas of nursing and surprise themselves by finding that they enjoy their work and learn a lot by doing it.

It is important that students be exposed to the many varieties of nursing work. Students are largely unaware of all of the specialties that exist, or could exist, other than that to which they have been exposed in school—namely, obstetrics, pediatrics, medical-surgical nursing, and psychiatric nursing. There is now provision for funding to increase options for nursing education to fill gaps in rural areas, with patients who have mental illness, and in other areas where nurses are needed (Indiana State Nurses Association, 2014). We can and should excite students about the fact that nurses belong everywhere and have the wherewithal to influence the quality of care in many different arenas.

Much of my scholarly research has been on nurses with disabilities. These nurses often leave nursing because they can no longer perform the physical tasks required or because they are pushed out by others who fear they will jeopardize patient safety. I and others have tried to advocate for admitting students with physical disabilities to nursing because there are so many areas of nursing work that don't require a lot of strength or the ability to lift or move swiftly. We continue to have shortages of nurses, but refuse to examine how we might retain nurses with disabilities or admit them to our programs. After all, we say we value critical thinking, but what we really seem to value is the physical ability to perform tasks.

Fragmentation of Nursing Education

Once again, the profession has determined to put its collective foot down about the entry level to professional practice. The Institute of Medicine (IOM, 2010) has recommended that 80% of nurses should have a baccalaureate degree by 2020 and that nurses should be able to transition seamlessly through the educational system to attain baccalaureate and graduate degrees, and schools of nursing are scrambling to develop and implement programs to make this happen. The American Nurses Association (ANA) has historically recommended and supported the BSN as the minimum degree required to practice professionally, yet today we still have multiple levels of entry.

Interestingly, the ANA welcomed the National Organization for Associate Degree Nursing as an affiliate member in December of 2013. "N-OADN promotes associate degree nursing through collaboration, advocacy and education to ensure excellence in the future of healthcare and professional nursing practice" (ANA, 2014, Jan/Feb). It is reasonable to be skeptical that we will be successful this time, especially because the factors that have prevented elimination of the diploma and associate degrees still remain in many parts of the country. What are the consequences if less than 80% of nurses have the BSN by 2020?

The Carnegie Foundation report (Benner, Sutphen, Leonard, & Day, 2010) concluded that our traditional pathways to becoming a nurse were not working. The report recommended changes that would enable nurses to advance through the levels of higher education more seamlessly, suggested that nursing education move away from a focus on skills toward requiring the knowledge that would be needed to practice effectively in the changing world of healthcare, and suggested that nurse residencies should be implemented more widely.

The survey data indicate that the vast majority of the respondents support the BSN as entry into practice. However, they differ with regard to how that should be enforced. Some say we should simply wipe out any vestige of associate degree and diploma programs. Others favor a stepwise approach that enables students—especially those with financial concerns—to obtain the BSN by moving seamlessly from an associate degree program or diploma school directly into the remaining classes. While in the minority among the respondents, some nurses ask that all three avenues to become an RN remain, and question why it is necessary to require the BSN. They put little faith and confidence in the Institute of Medicine Future of Nursing (2010) report.

If you reread Chapter 1, Chapter 2, and Chapter 3, it is possible to see how these varying levels of entry into practice developed and the purposes they served for the profession. However, it became clear early on that we should not be splintered and divided by "class"—and that is what varying degree levels do. One could argue that the elitism that has grown over time originally stemmed from the varying perspectives of nurses on the level of education they should receive.

Starting in the 1980s, there was a decline in the number of women choosing nursing as a profession, with a concomitant decline in students enrolling in BSN programs. This contributed to an increase in the average age of nurses and of nurse educators (Hahn, 2003). Many of these aging clinical nurses and nurse educators will soon retire. The DNP degree was not intended to prepare nurse educators, but we are using DNP graduates for that purpose to fill the gaps. In addition, we are offering every type of accelerated option possible for students to obtain undergraduate and graduate degrees to quickly fill the ranks of retiring nurses. Expediency seems to drive many nursing decisions, but as a result, we often sacrifice quality.

The Affordable Care Act has changed the healthcare landscape. This may make the difference regarding whether proposed changes in nursing actually occur this time. Nurses are seen to be vital to the changes taking place, and money is being made available to help educate nurses. In addition, nurses themselves seem to recognize that the BSN is necessary. Many students in associate degree programs acknowledge that they are pursuing the associate degree as an economical stepping stone to the baccalaureate. One often hears students in baccalaureate programs speak of going to graduate school, often bypassing the traditional rite of passage in a hospital clinical setting. Educational programs and difficulty finding hospital jobs has made graduate school a sooner rather than a later goal.

Have all of the varying tracks and programs diluted nursing education? Has there been a sacrifice of quality in the charge to attract people who want to be nurses in the quickest way possible? We shorten clinical time for students so we can shorten the length of their program. We allow undergraduate students to take graduate nursing courses before they have learned and practiced the fundamentals of nursing. We move graduate students through their programs quickly to put them in teaching and leadership positions before they are competent and confident regarding the basics of their new roles.

Ancillary Staff

Nursing has had an on-again, off-again relationship with ancillary personnel such as nurse's aides, medical assistants, licensed practical nurses, and others. At one time, the profession fought hard to prevent the introduction of registered care technicians. While the profession initially balked against having these additional personnel, once we realized that we didn't have enough nurses to complete every task and that nurses could perform aspects of care that would require more brain power than did changing a bed, we decided that as long as we could supervise those personnel, we would welcome their help. (Technically, in some states, nurses cannot supervise medical assistants, but in practice we do anyway). Over time, these personnel have gained ground with regard to the tasks they can perform and the responsibilities they have. While we have welcomed their help, we have complained to one another when the public cannot tell the difference between them and the registered nurse. Moreover, we have given tasks away that we should have retained.

Making a bed is not simply making a bed, it is an opportunity for the nurse to move the patient, examine the patient's skin, observe the patient, and talk to him or her.

Lately, we have begun to dedicate ourselves more directly to offering avenues to assist licensed practical nurses to gain entry into programs that will enable them to become registered nurses. I applaud this effort as long as we don't water down what is required to become an RN just to make sure that it is fast and easy. A great outcome could be the elimination of LPN programs so that when one refers to a nurse, they only mean a registered nurse. But if we lost LPNs, who would take their place? Do we need anyone to take their place? Should we return to a standardized uniform so the public can easily differentiate the RN from ancillary staff and other health professionals?

The DNP

Another nursing education issue that was clearly a hot button for survey respondents is the doctor of nursing practice (DNP) degree. In 2006, the DNP degree was considered by some to be "altering the landscape of nursing and health care" (Hathaway, Jacob, Stegbauer, Thompson, & Graff, 2006, p. 487). Others thought it developed naturally as a result of the NP programs that began in the 1960s (Hathaway et al., 2006). Case Western Reserve University started the first nursing practice doctorate (ND) in 1979. Meanwhile, NP programs evolved, and standardization took hold. Hathaway, *et al.* contend that the ND did not become standardized and that the DNP is the profession's answer to the need for a standardized practice doctorate. They also contend that because relatively few nurses are interested in pursuing PhD degrees but are interested in pursuing postmaster's education, the DNP is a reasonable option. Not only is the DNP not standardized, but more nurses are obtaining DNPs now than PhDs.

In 2005, the American Association of Colleges of Nursing (AACN) declared that preparation of advanced practice nurses would change from the master's degree to the DNP by 2015 (Nelson, 2005). Arguments against the DNP are refuted in detail in the Hathaway et al. paper, but do not address the public image of nursing with regard to its varying degrees, other than to admit that it can be daunting to try to explain our multiple entry-level programs to a high school senior contemplating whether to pursue nursing. The Hathaway et al. article smoothly dismisses objections that the DNP has less rigor than the PhD, and that the DNP dilutes the prestige of having a research doctorate. The public and our healthcare colleagues neither understand nor care about the differences among a PhD, EdD, DNSc, or DNP. They do not understand the nuances of having a practice doctorate that advances one's knowledge about quality improvement and expands the depth and breadth of clinical experience for APRNs. The public sees the myriad initials after our names, which even an experienced nurse academic and clinician cannot always decipher. When we attempt to explain, non-nurses' eyes glaze over, and one can easily read confusion on their faces.

It is interesting to note a comment by Marion et al. (2003) in their discussion of the DNP:

> The doctorates of nursing science (DNS/DNSc/DSN) and education (EdD) may have been intended to meet the need for advanced clinical practice and education, but a review of these programs reveals little difference between these and the research-intensive PhD programs. The nursing doctorate (ND), in contrast, has had clinical practice as its goal from its inception. However, the 4 existing ND programs are varied and lacking in a unified approach and have not created the critical mass needed for change at this time. (p. 2)

The public may value our ethics and trust us above all other professions, but they do not understand us. Perhaps we enjoy the mystery that surrounds nursing! We may kick and scream about the traditional image of female angels of mercy and ask to be valued for our ability to think critically and use sophisticated technology, but perhaps we enjoy the mystique we've cultivated by confusing the rest of the world about who we are and what we do. Patients simply want competent nurses who will provide excellent care and translate what doctors tell them into plain simple language. As a profession, we need people who can do that, as well as people who are current clinically and are aware of current research and how it can be used to improve patient care.

We want and need expert faculty to educate the newer generation of nurses. It doesn't seem to matter much anymore which doctoral degree faculty have because we are so desperate for nursing faculty. Certainly the DNP could have been the answer for us if education courses were a standard part of the curriculum. But wait, we have EdDs for that! We already had nurses who were educated to be educators. Now, we have created certification courses and new PhD programs to educate doctorally prepared nurses to be educators. This is long overdue. As a newly minted PhD, I was thrust into academic teaching with only one course (that I had chosen) in curriculum development under my belt. The assumption in nursing and some other disciplines has been that if you have a doctorate, you automatically know how to teach. Anyone who has taught, however, knows this is simply not true. One needs formal preparation to educate others in order to be an effective teacher.

The DNP has been lauded as the newest savior of nursing education and has been endowed with super powers that other degree programs have not achieved. Advances in technology, changes in healthcare, and workforce shortages have convinced us that the DNP is the answer. However, one need only look to the past as in the previous chapters to see that we frequently come up with a new idea and a new answer to the problems faced by healthcare and the profession, only to become disillusioned and have to develop a *new* new idea. Rather than adding to our repertoire of varying entry-level and graduate degrees, perhaps it's time to look at streamlining and enhancing the quality of programs in a few select areas. That stated, I think certain DNP programs prepare nurses with the expertise we need for the future in quality improvement, business, finance, leadership, and strategic planning. Soon, all nurses will need this knowledge in light of the changes occurring in healthcare.

Standardization of Nursing Education

Surprisingly, some nurse respondents commented that nursing education should be more standardized. This was not intended as an indictment of the fragmentation of nursing education in the form of varying entry-level degrees. Rather, it was a commentary on the different ways schools of nursing teach the required material. As mentioned, the survey responses are surprising because they indicate that not all schools emphasize topics that all nurses should know.

We are fortunate to have accrediting bodies that provide rigorous structure while also allowing programs to have some academic freedom in how they structure curricula. We must be wary of adopting a cookie-cutter approach to nursing education. Otherwise, we will be training technicians, rather than professionals, who cannot adapt their thinking or care to various populations or locales.

We do, however, need to standardize our approach to how we maintain rigor and whom we admit and graduate. Perhaps we should give more attention to cooperative relationships among schools as our nursing forebears suggested. They recommended that schools somehow alert one another if a nursing student failed, had integrity issues, or was otherwise unfit so that the student would not be considered for admission by other schools and could not ultimately become a nurse.

Men and Minorities

In 2003, nursing remained lacking in people of color and men (Hahn, 2003). In 2004, a survey of male nurses suggested that barriers to men in schools of nursing had barely changed and that the profession had done little to attract and retain men (O'Lynn, 2004). Gardner (2005) used phenomenology to explore the lived experiences of student nurses from racial and ethnic minorities. The themes that emerged from her research included feelings of loneliness and isolation, differentness, absence of acknowledgement or individuality from teachers, peers' lack of understanding and knowledge about cultural differences, coping with insensitivity and discrimination, desiring support from teachers, determination to build a better future, and overcoming obstacles. Gardner concluded that nurse educators should increase their awareness and knowledge regarding the needs, customs, and cultures of students from minority backgrounds.

Incivility and Professionalism

Several survey respondents mentioned continued bullying and the impact of incivility on students and the profession. Robertson (2012) reviewed the literature on incivility and found that "the additive effect of multiple aggravating factors threatens the viability of the educational process"

(p. 25). He concluded that students and faculty each think the other party is responsible and should resolve the problem. The American Nurses Association, along with other nursing organizations and the Joint Commission, have developed policies and resources aimed at reducing incivility in healthcare settings (Trossman, 2014).

Many survey respondents complained of the lack of professionalism displayed by students in clinical settings. According to these respondents, students dress inappropriately, wear gaudy jewelry, wear nail polish, display skin, and sport tattoos. In addition to inappropriate dress, they may speak disrespectfully to others, walk off the floor at inappropriate times, and badger faculty in the classroom. Students often expect immediate email responses from faculty, even at night and on weekends. They may line up outside of faculty offices to argue about test results and to question faculty expertise regarding a subject about which the student knows nothing.

There is no denying that students have become more vocal about what they like and don't like about the education they receive. This may be preferable to the old days, when students quaked in fear rather than asking a question of faculty or a superior. However, professionalism requires civility beginning in school. Incivility is unprofessional behavior, whether it's directed at a patient or faculty or staff at school or at a clinical site. Its presence or lack thereof should be graded, and that grade should weigh heavily when evaluating the student's readiness to enter the profession.

Faculty

While the profession recognizes the need to increase the nurse workforce, schools actively turn away a large number of potential students each year due to insufficient numbers of faculty, clinical placement sites, and budgets (www.aacn/nche.edu). According the AACN, schools find it hard to locate doctorally prepared faculty and have difficulty offering competitive salaries. In addition, schools must limit the number of students they accept because they don't have enough clinical sites at which to train them.

> Faculty members holding a junior rank as instructor or on a clinical track are more likely than associate profes-

sors or professors to move to different schools to assume full-time faculty positions or to leave for nonacademic nursing positions. Male faculty are more likely than female faculty to leave for full-time faculty positions at different schools, switch to part-time faculty positions, or leave for nonacademic nursing positions....The best predictor of faculty attritions is nontenure track/system status....In addition...having a doctoral degree increases the likelihood of switching to part-time faculty positions or leaving for nonacademic nursing positions. (Fang & Bednash, 2014, p. 172)

Programs that prepare nurse practitioners have also suffered due to lack of faculty as well as clinical sites and preceptors. This is due in part to faculty salaries being less than what a nurse practitioner educator might be paid working full-time clinically, the lack of doctorally prepared faculty, and the challenges faculty face to maintain their clinical practice hours while teaching and meeting faculty scholarship and committee expectations (Van Leuven, 2014). As the demand for NPs increases to meet the needs of primary care settings, in particular, new ways of developing clinical experiences for students will be necessary.

In the desperation to hire faculty, schools may hire people who have not practiced clinically in a long time, do not maintain a clinical practice, do not engage in scholarship, and have no teaching experience. We have now acknowledged that a doctoral degree does not a teacher make. Ideally, one should have classes in teaching to become an expert educator. However, many of us were hired in academe during a time when knowledge of nursing at a doctoral level was considered enough to be able to teach it.

Some schools are now offering doctorates and certificates in teaching to better prepare nurse educators. We have long allowed faculty to teach nursing without maintaining any clinical currency. How do we justify this? Some say teaching clinical courses keeps the educator current. However, there are many faculty who don't teach clinical classes and are still charged with educating students about cutting-edge medical and healthcare practices, diagnostics, and treatment. With regard to scholarship, unless someone teaches in a research institution, he or she may not participate in any accepted form of scholarship and still be employed. How can we pass on the importance of scholarship and research to our students if we don't engage in it ourselves? There are so many ways to be scholarly, there really is no excuse now for faculty to not engage in some form of scholarship.

Clinical faculty also may be lacking in current clinical skills and yet are responsible for teaching students how to practice competently. Conversely, nursing staff working full time in care settings may be asked to teach when they have no background or training in education.

Clinical Education

Nurses who responded to our survey were vehement in their concern about the number of hours and quality of clinical experiences nursing students receive, claiming they are inadequate to prepare nurses for the realities of the real world. Interestingly, while we all agree that clinical practica are vital to learning how to become a nurse, we know little about the best practices of teaching and learning that help students learn what they need to know to be safe and knowledgeable clinicians (Ironside, McNelis, & Ebright, 2014). Using a multimethod design, researchers studied three schools of nursing of different types and from different regions within the U.S. to observe and record students and faculty during clinical practica. In total, 30 students and six faculty were involved in the study. The study found that "the traditional focus on task completion persists and consumes (and may often be at odds with) students' learning in practice settings" (Ironside et al., 2014, p. 189). Despite our recognition as a profession that the nurse must be able to think critically, problem solve, and practice holistically, the focus in the actual clinical setting is still on whether the student can perform tasks. "Continuing to structure students' clinical experiences around the provision of routine care is insufficient because students miss important information and the more subtle cues inherent in actual clinical situations" (p. 190).

Clinical sites are in short supply for entry-level nursing students and APRN students. Service learning has been proposed as a way to provide additional opportunities for nurse practitioner students to gain experience in primary care. "Service learning is a structured learning experience combining community service with preparation and reflection" (Sheikh, 2014, p. 354). Service learning incorporates community service with didactic learning, good citizenship, socialization into the advanced practice role, and new skills.

Interprofessional Education

Historically, we have had tension in physician-nurse relationships. New nurses still struggle with how to talk to physicians and work collaboratively. However, rather than dwell on difficulties with individual physicians, both the medical and nursing professions—as well as other health professionals—are working to increase interprofessional (IP) collaboration.

Learning from students in other healthcare disciplines is more reflective of the reality of working in most healthcare settings because now more than ever, professionals have to work as a team to provide high-quality, cost-effective, efficient care. However, faculty from each of the healthcare disciplines were not educated in an interprofessional environment, so they may lack the skills to train students appropriately (Becker, Hanyok, & Walton-Moss, 2014). Becker et al. (2014) refer to the preconceptions faculty have regarding IP education as "turf and baggage" (p. 240). Turf issues refer to conflicts between and among professional organizations. Baggage refers to the preconceived ideas each discipline brings to the table. Physicians have traditionally thought of themselves as being in charge with the ultimate responsibility for the patient, and the nurse was expected to execute physician orders. Tension has developed to a boiling point since the advent of the APRN and subsequent conflicts regarding scope of practice. The Affordable Care Act has exacerbated the problem (Becker et al., 2014).

I have interviewed applicants to medical school and have spoken with young medical students and physicians, and I am impressed with their verbal commitment to interprofessional team work. I believe they can really change the physician-nurse relationship for the better. Other healthcare disciplines also seem committed to working collegially instead of competitively, so I am hopeful that concerns about status will eventually dissipate. Interprofessional educational opportunities are needed to ensure this, however. If students become accustomed to working together to solve problems and manage patient cases, then they will readily adapt to doing so, and doing it better than we do now, when they graduate.

Not every school—very few in fact—has the resources on campus to enable interprofessional experiences among the health professions. It becomes quite challenging when the campus does not include a medical school, health professions school, and a nursing school. However, partnerships with healthcare agencies and other universities can help provide opportunities. In addition, nursing students don't have to necessarily partner with other students in the health professions to learn how to work interprofessionally. Attending classes that are team taught by nursing and faculty from the school of education or the college of arts and sciences, for example, can provide opportunities to learn how disciplines interact. Carefully crafted class exercises and assignments can help students understand how to communicate with someone who doesn't speak their professional language, resolve conflicts, and manage personnel and other issues that can arise in any profession.

It is important to mention the influx of military veterans on college campuses and the positive impact this can have on student learning. Military veterans often bring maturity, experience, and a worldview to class that are foreign to young undergraduate students. As active-duty service people, veterans were expected to leave their biases behind and work with people from all over the United States and other countries, follow orders, question but behave respectfully when interacting with authority figures, and produce high-quality work. Nursing students can surely learn from their example.

Conclusion

It is apparent that we must align our actions with our hopes for the future as we consider what is next for nursing education. We must, once and for all, try to unify to correct our past mistakes instead of creating new programs and ideas to fill the gaps that have resulted. Let's truly make the BSN required for entry into practice or else restructure the DNP to become an entry-level degree for everyone. Let's eliminate the LPN, associate degree, and diploma so that we can say that all novice RNs are prepared at the same level. We've claimed we would do this throughout our history, but we find excuses for not seeing it through. Frequently, economic forces get in the way. Let's also agree to be selective about whom we admit and whom we allow to graduate. This will not jeopardize tuition and student numbers because many more will want to become nurses if they respect our value as professionals rather than see us as technicians or as unskilled.

KEY POINTS ABOUT THE FUTURE OF NURSING EDUCATION

Critical thinking

Rigor

Broad liberal education

Community nursing care

Nursing specialties

Fragmentation of nursing education

Ancillary staff

The DNP

Standardization of nursing education

Men and minorities

Incivility and professionalism

Faculty issues

Clinical education

Interprofessional education

References

American Nurses Association. (2014, Jan/Feb). ANA welcomes the National Organization for Associate Degree Nursing. *The American Nurse, 5.*

Becker, K. L., Hanyok, L. A., & Walton-Moss, B. (2014). The turf and baggage of nursing and medicine: Moving forward to achieve success in inter-professional education. *The Journal for Nurse Practitioners, 10*(4), 240–244.

Benner, P., Sutphen, M., Leonard, V., & Day, L. (2010). *Educating nurses: A call for radical transformation.* San Francisco: Jossey-Bass.

Fang, D., & Bednash, G. (2014). Attrition of full-time faculty from schools of nursing with baccalaureate and graduate programs, 2010 to 2011. *Nursing Outlook, 62*(3), 164–173.

Gardner, J. (2005). Barriers influencing the success of racial and ethnic minority students in nursing programs. *Journal of Transcultural Nursing, 16*(2), 155–162.

Hahn, J. (2003). The federal budget and the impact on nursing education, research, and innovative practice. *Newborn and Infant Nursing Reviews, 3*(1), 5–10.

Hathaway, D., Jacob, S., Stegbauer, C., Thompson, C., & Graff, C. (2006). The practice doctorate: Perspectives of early adopters. *Journal of Nursing Education, 45*(12), 487–496.

Im, E-O., & Chang, S. J. (2012). Current trends in nursing theories. *The Journal of Nursing Scholarship, 44*(2), 156–164.

Indiana State Nurses Association. (2014, February/March). Independent study: The evolving practice of nursing. *ISNA Bulletin,* 7–10.

Institute of Medicine (2010). The future of nursing: Leading change, advancing health. Washington, DC: The National Academies Press.

Ironside, P. M., McNelis, A. M., & Ebright, P. (2014). Clinical education in nursing; Rethinking learning in practice settings. *Nursing Outlook, 62*(3), 185–191.

Marion, L., Viens, D., O'Sullivan, A. L., Crabtree, K., Fontana, S., & Price, M. M. (2003). The practice doctorate in nursing: Future or fringe. *Topics in Advanced Practice Nursing eJournal, 3*(2), 1–8.

Neal-Boylan, L. (2013). *The nurse's reality gap: Overcoming barriers between academic achievement and clinical success.* Indianapolis, IN: Sigma Theta Tau Publishing.

Neal-Boylan, L. J. (2008). *On becoming a home health nurse: Practice meets theory in home care nursing.* Washington, DC: Home Care University and Home Health Nursing Association.

Nelson, R. (2005). AJN Reports: is there a doctor in the house? *The American Journal of Nursing, 105*(5), 28–29.

O'Lynn, C. E. (2004). Gender-based barriers for male students in nursing education programs: Prevalence and perceived importance. *Journal of Nursing Education, 43*(5), 229–236.

Policy brief: Home Health Care Planning Act of 2013 (H. R. 2504, S. 1332). (2014). Retrieved from www.aacn.nche.edu

Robertson, J. E. (2012). Can't we all just get along? *Incivility Research, 33*(1), 21–26.

Sheikh, K. R. (2014). Expanding clinical models of nurse practitioner education: Service learning as a curricular strategy. *The Journal for Nurse Practitioners, 19*(5), 352–356.

Trossman, S. (2014, Jan/Feb). Toward civility: ANA, nurses promote strategies to prevent disruptive behaviors. *The American Nurse, 46*(1), 6.

Van Leuven, K. A. (2014). Preparing the next generation of nurse practitioners. *The Journal for Nurse Practitioners, 10*(4), 271–276.

Chapter 8

Looking Toward the Future for Nursing Practice

Bea, the special duty nurse, couldn't be there today. "Could you sit with Mr. Farber for an hour?" the doctor had asked me. He told me to call him if need be, and he'd come and pronounce the patient dead.

I scrambled around for a uniform, finding a crumpled dress in my "winter drawer." It smelled of cedar and cigarettes from my husband's sweaters. It was a bit old fashioned, but Mr. Farber certainly wouldn't care. My organdy cap needed no inspection, however. A cherished possession earned after all of the vicissitudes of nurse's training, it was not yet an anachronism. It was a cap of linen with a black ribbon on the edge. The cap, which I had perched tentatively on my head, was emblematic of my status as a registered nurse.

This was 1958, and nursing was almost entirely a profession of women. I wanted to go sit with Mr. Farber and ease his dying moments. My neighbors would watch the children until my husband got home, and he would give them dinner. "Must she nurse everyone in Brooklyn and run every time someone calls?" I could just hear my husband saying this when he arrived home to find me gone. But he was proud, too. I was the neighbor with the magical qualities. I could "make it better," just as my mother had done many years before.

A cab took me to the large teaching hospital nearby—the place where I had played in the emergency room as a toddler while waiting for my mother to finish work as the charge nurse. I would roll myself in bandages and sniff the disinfectant and elixirs in heavy little glass bottles. I would grind the glass stoppers as I removed them, enjoying the crunching sound while hoping they wouldn't break, and use the stoppers to place scent behind my ears, the way our upstairs tenant did when putting on her makeup. At dusk, my mother and I would walk home along the streetcar tracks. I would smell quite awful but feel very happy.

When I arrived at the hospital, I met Mr. Farber's wife outside his private room. She extended her hand and a $50 bill to me, but I told her I wouldn't accept it. We entered the room together. Mr. Farber was nearly invisible behind the heavy cellophane oxygen tent that was draped at his sides and tucked into the bedding. A lime green oxygen tank stood beside the bed. I scanned the room for a "no smoking" sign and felt reassured that it was posted beside the bed.

I introduced myself to the patient and reminded him that we had met once before at his cousin's wedding. He didn't respond, but I sensed that he understood. Before I had a chance to assess Mr. Farber further, his wife asked me to step into the hall to meet their best friends. I was annoyed by the distraction and had already placed the stethoscope to my ears, but removed it and followed her out of the room. Seated on the steps of an old metal staircase the staff seldom used were a man and a woman of indeterminate age. I hardly noticed the woman because the man was in tears. "Nurse," he said, "please don't let Joe die on me. We've been together since Anzio."

I sent the three to have coffee in the hospital cafeteria and went to the nurse's station to confer with the nurse on duty:

"Blood pressure and pulse have been very erratic," she said as we walked down the corridor. "He had a massive heart attack. Just stay with him, it won't be long now." Back in his room, I opened the zipper of the oxygen tent and I placed the blood pressure cuff on Mr. Farber's—Joe's—arm. His blood pressure was OK—not great, but within normal limits. So too were his pulse and respirations. I repeated this every 15 minutes and then every half hour since there was no change. His wife brought coffee and a sandwich for me and lightly waved to Joe before going home with her friends to rest.

The doctor called me at the nurse's station at about 10 p.m. "Is it over yet? I really need to call it a day," he said wearily. "No, it's not over," I said. "He's improving! His vital signs are stable. This man is not going to die today—not for quite a while, I think. I am going to give the charge nurse report and go home."

Bea called me three days later to thank me for covering for her. "Joe wants to know where his angel is. He says you certainly looked like an angel with a cap through that tent. He's out of bed and in the chair today without oxygen." Later that day, she called again to tell me that Joe's good friend and Army buddy had dropped dead on the way to the hospital to visit him. I was horrified. The stress his friend had been going through had gone completely unnoticed by all of us.

Several factors have influenced the changes that have occurred in nursing practice since 2000. These factors include advances in technology, changes in reimbursement and funding practices, new legislation, and an increased variety of educational programs offered. There is more emphasis on the quality and continuity of care and on providing care by the appropriate staff in the appropriate setting (Indiana State Nurses Association, 2014).

The Affordable Care Act (ACA) is intended to emphasize disease prevention and increased use of primary care and community health services. Nurses, long accustomed to educating patients, must now understand the financial implications of various healthcare services and help their patients make informed decisions. Nurses are also used to working in teams and may be more likely to lead teams of other professionals to help prevent hospital admissions and readmissions. Technology, including electronic medical records, telehealth, and tools used to explore the impact of genetics and genomics on diagnosis and treatment, has required the nurse to become more familiar with informatics. Changes in funding and reimbursement require more accountability from inpatient facilities and their staff, including nurses.

Many of the issues raised by survey respondents and in today's literature echo those from bygone days of nursing. Relationships with physicians in the practice setting, particularly for new nurses, remain a problem, as does bullying and burnout. Nurses report elitism and disunity in the profession, unacceptable working conditions, burdensome workloads, inadequate pay, a confused public image of nurses, and the use and misuse of ancillary staff.

Care-delivery models are changing, and nursing is being redefined. The nursing shortage continues, and more nurses are needed to move into community settings to practice. Nurses may be choosing high technology interventions over the basics of nursing care. There are not enough jobs for new RNs, and standardized residencies and orientations are necessary to ease the transition into practice. Communication, collaboration, and professionalism are suffering. Disaster preparedness, while a significant part of nursing in the form of preparation for war and the aftermath of war, has taken on new meanings since 9/11.

Relationships With Physicians

While physicians may acknowledge that there is a shortage of their kind practicing in primary care, and although many (privately) acknowledge the quality of care provided by APRNs, they remain publicly skeptical of the ability of nurse practitioners to fill their shoes. The American Medical Association has been vocal in warning the public about the differences between NPs and physicians, and has made a point of highlighting the variations in educational preparation. While they may say we should all work together in teams, they espouse that the physician should lead the team (Iglehart, 2013).

Clearly, physicians as a group (with some exceptions) still see themselves as superior to nurses. This may never change. However, individuals and pockets of physicians do express respect for what nurses do and are willing to work together and with other professionals. It is important as we move into the future and the changing healthcare landscape that physicians not only give lip service to interprofessional team work, but internalize it. Perhaps they should look at how poorly their efforts at superiority have worked in the past and embrace what everyone else has been doing with the common goal of high-quality care delivery.

Bullying and Incivility

Nurses continue to encounter incivility, most often in the form of verbal abuse, in the work setting. There is a correlation between this abuse and patient safety (Budin, Brewer, Chao, & Kovner, 2013). A survey of 1,407 early-career RNs found that almost half of these nurses had experienced verbal abuse, mostly in the form of being ignored or spoken to condescendingly. These nurses were most often Caucasian, married, generally healthy, and not currently enrolled in school. Most were native English speakers and worked in a hospital doing 12-hour shift work. The researchers recommend "evidence-based strategies that address the problems inherent with verbal abuse from nurse colleagues" (Budin et al., 2013, p. 314) and suggest structured training in communication, conflict resolution, and assertiveness (Budin et al., 2013).

I think that although new nurses are most often the target (Budin et al., 2013) of verbal abuse, they may also display behaviors that encourage frustration on the part of their more experienced colleagues. This is not to in any way suggest that they or anyone else deserves to be mistreated; however, given the attitudes that nursing faculty often encounter from students, it is not a stretch to assume that these attitudes are carried over into the work setting after graduation.

Students can be abusive and demanding of faculty. They may come to class unprepared, miss class, or miss clinical days, but still expect good grades. Students often have their parents call and bully faculty and administrators. Students who are not respectful and are demanding and intransigent while in school are not likely to be humble when beginning their first job. Experienced nurses may be on the defensive when encountering new graduates based on past behavior, or they may be reactive when a new graduate adopts an attitude of entitlement when they know essentially nothing about actual nursing. Of course, there are people who are simply mean and may resent the intrusion of new graduates.

We should nurture our new nurses and adopt the attitude of *esprit de corps* from days of old in nursing. However, new graduates must do their part and come to school and work prepared, without the expectation that others will solve their problems for them. This, again, is where critical thinking plays a significant role in nursing practice. If a student is accustomed to having every need met, then where is the incentive to learn how to solve one's own problems?

Workload and Burnout

Several nurse respondents mentioned self-care and the need for work-life balance. Nurses both in academe and in practice report little time or energy for life outside of work. I have written about "nurse heroics" (Neal-Boylan, 2012) in the context of nurses with disabilities. We are ingrained with the obligation to be available and ready to fulfill every patient need during every waking moment. Nurses rarely take their breaks or mealtimes in part because they feel obligated to be present, but also because they are wary of how other nurses will view them if they leave. While "presence" is an integral part of nursing care, we need to trust our colleagues to cover for us so we can restore ourselves. Nurses with disabilities have conveyed that if they take a sick day or take a break to rest, even though they are entitled to these opportunities, they are considered shirkers. Florence Nightingale (1860) encouraged nurses to take time to rejuvenate, writing that one could not care for others well if she did not care for herself.

Susan Trossman (2014, p. 1) says that because nurses and females are nurturers, we give until our own well-being suffers. It is important that we review our schedules, learn to say no, set limits, and turn off communication technology when we are not working. Time-outs, breaks, vacations, and exercise are other strategies suggested by nurses in Trossman's article.

I hear a lot about how hard nurse educators work. I know this from personal experience. But I also know that professionals in other disciplines work just as hard. Nurse academics are expected to teach a full load, participate on committees, keep current clinically, and maintain a program of scholarship. If one wants to also have a life outside of work, this becomes a tremendous challenge. I think the profession should help nurse academics and clinical nurses learn more about time management. It's not something we teach sufficiently in schools of nursing. We may suggest that students learn how to balance work and life activities, but we are generally not doing enough to teach them techniques for doing this. If they have to care for several patients at once while in school, they may, of necessity, have to learn to balance priorities. But, we have to improve on this ourselves before we can be of much help to students.

I think it is wonderful that many in the profession are calling more attention to the need for self-care. However, hard work and sacrifice are as old as nursing itself. My grandmother worked 12-hour shifts, 5 or 6 days per week in the 1920s and 1930s. She and her colleagues picketed for 8-hour days. We like to think that we work harder than ever today or have more demands on our time. But in fact, the nurses of yesteryear did not have the time-saving technology that we have now. My grandmother had to sterilize the glass syringe and needle she carried with her between patients. She and my mother, who was also a nurse, had to prepare meals for patients as part of patient care. There are many things earlier generations of nurses had to do that we no longer need to do. To be sure, some new tasks have supplanted those responsibilities, but careful analysis reveals that earlier generations managed to do more with less. We like to see ourselves as martyrs to some extent (myself included). I don't think our emphasis on long hours and self-sacrifice can even begin to lessen until we have enough nurses to care for our patients safely and we give permission to one another to care for ourselves.

Pay and Poor Working Conditions

In general, nurse respondents reported difficult working conditions. This problem seems to be pervasive across settings. Many also said that nurses are paid poorly or unfairly and that there should be a differential between the associate degree-prepared nurse and the baccalaureate-prepared nurse. There were many comments about unionization and how this should be eliminated because it does not serve the nurse well.

Nurses continue to be responsible for several complicated patient cases, particularly in inpatient settings. This jeopardizes safety and makes the nurse liable even though the expectations are unreasonable. The issue of too many patients to one nurse has long been a problem in nursing, going back to having student nurses run the hospital during the night shift. However, if there is a nursing shortage and/or if organizations are unwilling or unable to pay for RNs, then the nurse is put in charge of more patients than anyone can reasonably manage. We must continue to rail against this practice, but not settle for an increase in the use of ancillary staff to relieve our workloads.

Back to Basics

Many nurses who responded to the survey described the loss of "back to basics" nursing care. They claimed that nurses do not provide basic care anymore, such as bathing, ambulation, IV care, etc. While none seem to regret the advances in technology that save lives and often enhance nurse efficiency, they worry that these basics of care are being passed on to ancillary staff. Nurses "who have been around" and were educated to provide the basics remember learning that "AM care" was an opportunity to talk to the patient and conduct a thorough assessment. As another example, emptying the urinary catheter was an opportunity to examine the color of the urine, its consistency, and odor, as well as the volume.

We have given many tasks to ancillary staff because of our time constraints and our need to focus on activities that require critical analysis. However, electronic health records often prevent us from looking at the patient while we take a history or actually examining the patient instead of relying on the previous nurse's notes. I experienced this with my own father, who was discharged to a rehabilitation facility after a long hospitalization. When I went to see him for the first time, I helped him get out of bed to go to the dining room. He was sleepy in bed because he was given much more of a medication than he ever took at home. This resulted in the LPNs (who provided all of the care, along with nurse's aides) to leave him in bed and delay his lunch and any opportunity to go to physical therapy or to ambulate.

When I got him up, I helped to dress him. Seating him on the edge of the bed, I noticed a huge hematoma all along one side of his back.

The nurses denied that he had fallen. No one had looked at his back or at his chart, which clearly stated that he was taking a blood thinner. No one had alerted the physician or checked his blood levels. An RN would have understood the implications of the medications and their dosages on his level of awareness, would have looked at his skin and noted the hematoma, and would have connected it with his anticoagulant. This is not an isolated example, but exemplary of what happens in many settings in which non-RNs provide most of the "basic" care and RNs are too removed from the assessment of the patient.

Elitism

Interestingly, elitism seems to have been a problem in nursing since the profession's early days. Nurses caring for patients considered nursing leaders to be too far removed from actual clinical practice to be able to understand their needs. This perception has continued, and is clearly alive and well today. Additionally, the perception of disunity has grown. Nurses feel that we are separated from one another with regard to educational background, professional organizations (which compete against each other for membership and resources), work setting, and job title.

Survey respondents asked that nursing faculty keep current clinically and that nursing administrators be willing and able to "get their hands dirty" in clinical settings. Many nurses feel that we dismiss bedside nursing as being performed by nurses who are either new to nursing and going through the rites of passage or who cannot, for whatever reason, go on to graduate school to move away from the bedside. How did we get to a point of conveying that the nurse at the bedside was somehow deficient or incapable of "professional" or leadership status? In public, we may laud their work and expertise, and find ourselves supremely grateful to them when they are caring for our own loved ones. But among ourselves, we whisper that nurses must go on for higher education.

Nurses who care for patients embody what nursing is in the public view. The public trusts nurses because of the "bedside" nurse who cares for their mother or child. We are fooling ourselves if we think the public trusts nurses above other professionals because they admire our educators or our researchers. The public sees nurses at the bedside and the immediate difference they make. They don't see the impact of nurse educators or researchers except very indirectly.

Clearly, nurses who provide direct care full time feel that they are viewed as somehow inferior to nurses with graduate degrees or in leadership positions. If we want RNs to continue to provide care to patients, then we must show appreciation for the nurses who perform that care. Otherwise, we could have LPNs and nurse's aides, as well as other health professionals, take over the care of our patients so all nurses can be administrators, professors, and researchers. I don't think this is what we want, but we talk out of both sides of our mouths. Yes, nurses should have at least a baccalaureate degree, but must they get a graduate degree to work to the fullest extent of their ability? If we make a revamped and reconfigured DNP the practice doctorate as entry into practice and eliminate other entry-level degrees, the RN will be prepared to care for patients at the bedside and also have a working knowledge of all of the areas they will need to know to practice in the future.

We could fit into the DNP curriculum all the material a nurse needs to know to keep up with a changing healthcare system, including the basics such as pediatric and adult care (with added emphasis on community and mental-health nursing), but with the addition of genomics, informatics, infectious disease, economics, business, global health, quality improvement, and other topics. A practice doctorate for entry into the profession is not unreasonable, given that physical therapists now require a doctorate and occupational therapists have moved in that direction. No one could look down upon a nurse regardless of what he or she chooses to do because we would all have respect for each other's foundational knowledge and skills. We could eliminate our preconceived ideas and prejudices about what each of us knows because the foundation would not only be the same, but be comprehensive and futuristic. We could eliminate public confusion about who is a nurse and what a nurse knows.

Academics and researchers could still obtain an EdD or PhD. Nurses interested in being clinical leaders would still have myriad options from which to choose, such as the clinical nurse leader or the advanced practice registered nurse.

As things are now, there are so many roles in nursing extant and yet to be created that if a nurse with a BSN does not want to get a graduate degree, why should we pressure him or her to do so? I have seen so many students who apply for nurse practitioner programs who have no inkling what an NP actually does. Students are often encouraged to bypass clinical practice and go straight into a graduate program or to apply for graduate school when they don't know what they really want to do in nursing. But when we do this, we shoot ourselves in the foot. We develop nurses with graduate degrees when we might not have jobs for them, and we expose the profession to further loss of educated nurses who become frustrated doing jobs for which they have no passion. As in days of old, these disillusioned nurses are likely to denigrate the profession to their friends and discourage them from becoming nurses.

Disunity

Nursing organizations should unite. The ANA is clearly making an effort to do this, and has many affiliate organizations (ANA, 2014, p. 5). The ANA has also undergone restructuring in recognition of the fragmentation of nursing's voice and the reduction in membership that has taken place over the years.

It is important that we make nursing organizations, journal subscriptions, and nursing conferences affordable and accessible for all nurses. Many are so cost prohibitive, only nurse academics, administrators, or researchers can afford to belong or attend. Consequently, important information is not conveyed to all nurses, and nursing leaders are not exposed to points of view from the nurses who actually care for patients.

I think the inability to attend conferences or afford organization memberships also accounts for the variations in the survey responses regarding what is happening in nursing. Clearly, nurses are not all getting the same messages about what is happening in the profession, so it is difficult to speak with one voice.

Public Image

Although nursing is a profession highly trusted by the public, many nurse respondents remarked that our image badly needs restoration. As described in Chapter 7, "Looking Toward the Future for Nursing

Education," nurses decry the appearances of both nursing students (in clinical settings) and nurses. Visible tattoos, fake and long nails, excess makeup, body piercings, and long-hanging hair does not convey professionalism. I have noticed that nurses don't always put their hair up when caring for patients. Not only is this unsanitary for the patient, it also exposes the nurse to bacteria. Some nurses recommend going back to a standardized uniform that would eliminate these unprofessional aspects and also make us more recognizable to the public.

Ancillary Staff

The issue of if and how ancillary staff is utilized to assist nurses or augment care delivery has been discussed throughout this book, starting in Chapter 1, "Nurses Are Made Not Born: Educational Reform Frames the Profession (1900–1935)." The problem continues to exist. Throughout our history, nurses have frequently won battles against others who would replace us with unlicensed healthcare workers. However, over time, we have given away bit by bit aspects of care that were once the purview of RNs. We continue to have LPNs in many settings. If we were more united as a profession, we would be more empowered to fight encroachment on our turf.

This may seem contradictory to what I wrote earlier about being more interprofessional. However, preventing others from doing nursing work is not counter to being interprofessional. We cannot allow others to undervalue us and therefore pay others less to do what requires the expertise and skill of an RN. It is time we eliminated the LPN role. Offering programs aimed at helping LPNs return to school for RN education is one approach, but only if we don't water down what they need to know in an attempt to make education more convenient or expeditious. The culture change between LPN and RN is key to making someone an RN. Simply giving them the classes and clinical hours they did not receive in the LPN program is not sufficient.

With the ongoing nursing shortage, the problem of nurses performing tasks they are not licensed to perform is also an issue (Lubbe & Roets, 2014). This problem may be more common outside of the United States, but its existence warrants our attention as we plan for the future.

In the future, nursing roles are likely to morph and change. Nurses must have the final say as to how this happens. We must unite our organizations and our efforts to present a strong voice, and recruit physicians and other healthcare professionals to support our efforts to maintain the core values and purposes of the profession.

Care Delivery

Despite the ongoing controversies faced by NPs as we try to solidify the Consensus Model and erase supervisory and collaborative agreements, we have made great strides in expanding health care-delivery services through nurse-managed health clinics (Title III of the Public Health Service Act-http://legcounsel.house.gov/Comps/PHSA_CMD.pdf). APRNs manage these clinics and work with other disciplines to deliver high-quality primary care (http://www.nncc.us/site/).

As the population ages, the demand for nursing-home care is increasing. Residents require more services due to age and frailty. Those who can go back to or remain in the community are being cared for using home-health or other community-living options (Castle, 2008; Zhang, Unruh, & Wan, 2013). A study by Zhang et al. (2013) concluded that current nurse staffing in nursing homes is insufficient to meet the needs of the increasing nursing-home resident population and that government support is needed to increase reimbursement to help reduce gaps and improve efficiency.

We need to staff nursing homes with more RNs and decrease our reliance on LPNs and nurse's aides. Nursing homes are not warehouses for our aged and infirm. Residents should receive the best care possible. Nursing-home owners have long been unwilling to pay for RNs. This continues to sacrifice quality and safety. The majority of the public does not know how to differentiate quality long-term care. It is our job to educate them.

Rutherford (2012) discussed the longstanding tradition of billing nursing services in the hospital under "room and board." She claims that we are too focused on whether the current system reflects the value of nursing, but not focused enough on identifying "nursing revenue as a value driver" (p. 196) and a way to "justify an investment in the profession" (p. 199). Rutherford's comments reflect changes happening in healthcare. We must become more business and finance savvy so that we are not at the mercy of others who determine what our services are worth. We need more nurses in the boardrooms of both healthcare and non-healthcare organizations so we can influence healthcare delivery and policy that affects healthcare.

Insufficient Jobs

Nurses who responded to the survey confirmed what new nurses have said about the difficulty finding jobs right out of nursing school (Neal-Boylan, 2013). For many years, new graduates had many offers. Today, however, it takes longer to get a job in an acute-care setting. Many hospitals want experienced nurses, partly because residencies and internships can be expensive. It is important to help new graduates understand that nursing experience in other settings is not only very valuable, but also "counts" as nursing. If we increase our emphasis on nursing in community settings while students are still in school, they will be better prepared for these jobs and have a greater appreciation for the services they can provide outside of the hospital.

Residencies and Orientations, Preceptors, and Mentors

Nurse residencies and internships, as well as strong and knowledgeable preceptors and mentors, can significantly affect the transition of new RNs and APRNs into practice. In its 2010 report, the Institute of Medicine (IOM) supported the need for residencies for all new nurses. Schools of nursing appear to be working to develop partnerships with clinical agencies to implement these programs. However, they remain without standardization (Barnett, Minnick, & Norman, 2014) and probably will for some time.

Barnett et al. (2014) conducted a survey of hospitals, and 198 responded. According to their findings, the residency programs differed with regard to length, but most often began with less emphasis on direct care of patients, which increased during the residency.

> New nurse graduates and their mentors should understand that the content and structure of all nursing residencies are not the same nor are all implemented with the same labor inputs...When making a decision about which, if any, NRP [nurse residency program] to select, the new nurse should consider the number of residents entering and completing the program, the ratio of mentors to residents, activities, project requirements, and opportunities for career planning. (Barnett et al. 2014, p. 182–183)

A solid and lengthy orientation or residency is especially important for new graduates so they can develop confidence in their new role and others can rely on their competence. These orientations and residencies should become more standardized by setting. In other words, acute care hospitals should settle on a standardized curriculum and length of orientation and train and incentivize their preceptors. Additional information specific to each organization must be included, but the basics needed to work in acute care should be reviewed. Nurses starting out in home care or public health should receive 9 months to a year of consistent precepting as well as orientation about the unique aspects of home health or public health nursing.

Experienced nurses who move into new jobs also need good orientations and precepting or mentoring for their own sake and that of their patients. Many nurses who are experienced RNs but who returned for graduate degrees reenter the workforce in entirely new roles. While they are not beginners, they certainly require a period of familiarization.

Communication and Collaboration

Nurse respondents acknowledged that there is value in giving the direct-care nurse some time to perform administrative duties, and for administrators to perform some direct-care tasks. Both parties should understand what the other does and how they contribute to the organization. In addition, more opportunities for inter-professional teamwork should be provided in the clinical setting, such as interdisciplinary rounding and conferencing. Include representatives from all healthcare disciplines in discussions of ethical dilemmas and patient issues. A chance to observe someone from another discipline as that person goes about his or her work could help to inform the nurse of who best to utilize for the good of the patient, and can also increase appreciation for how that discipline contributes to the care of the patient.

In addition, observing a nurse from within the continuum of care but in a setting different from one's own can help nurses plan care. I once taught a graduate class of all acute-care nurses. I exposed them to home healthcare experiences. They were shocked, despite years of experience in nursing, at how hard it actually is for patients to implement what we teach them in inpatient settings when they arrive home. They vowed to plan future care and discharges with the home setting in mind.

In addition, previous generations of nurses and other professionals can provide insight into how elders might perceive the care they receive. They have the perspective of both a healthcare professional and an older person with illness or disability. Taking advantage of their experiences can lend insight into how to provide better care.

Professionalism

Professionalism (or lack thereof) may mean different things to different people. However, it was a common topic among nurse respondents. Nurses lament the lack of a unified professional image and the public's confusion over who the nurse is. But the concern goes beyond this to a lack of pride in appearance and comportment and a disregard for both common courtesies and professional etiquette.

Nurses often set a poor example by displaying the same poor health behaviors about which we chide our patients, such as smoking, drug and alcohol use, and obesity. We want the public to differentiate the RN from the LPN, nurse's aide, or housekeeping staff. Therefore, we should set ourselves above others in our professional appearance, with all due respect to our coworkers. If we present a disorderly or unprofessional appearance, then it is a logical jump to think we may be disorganized and incapable.

Disaster Preparedness

The first three chapters of this book discussed how the nursing profession struggled with ways to prepare nurses to care for soldiers and the public during wartime and in the aftermath of war. While this remains a topic today for nurses serving in military hospitals, units in settings of war, and nurses who care for veterans, there is less emphasis in the general nursing literature on how to prepare the profession to go to war. Since September 11, 2001, there has been increasing emphasis on disaster preparedness and managing bioterrorism events. Disasters are increasingly prevalent and stem from global unrest, climate change, population changes, and new infections (Baack & Alfred, 2013). The demand for nursing increases with these events (Baack & Alfred, 2013; Lavin, 2006).

> Not only must nurses be prepared to respond to major disasters to meet the needs of those affected, but they must also possess the knowledge needed for management of patients with special needs, such as the elderly, children, persons with mobility impairments, and even persons with mental health issues. (Baack & Alfred, 2013, p. 282)

I think there was a lot of emphasis on disaster preparedness in the early years of the new millennium, but the emphasis has since waxed and waned depending on what is happening domestically and around the world. It is important that nurses receive consistent reminders about how to manage themselves and others in the event of a disaster. Also, shootings in schools and public places have increased. Nurses should have a large role in educating the public to protect their safety and in providing mental health care and general healthcare to victims and families.

Conclusion

Sweeping changes are occurring in healthcare, and the landscape promises to look very different for healthcare providers in every discipline. Nursing can lead the way and model for others what we have known how to do for a very long time. Nurses have long worked in teams and have coordinated care for patients. Physicians consider the advent of the patient-centered medical home, for example, to be a new concept, when it is really basically a restructuring of the case-management models with which nurses are very familiar. The idea of working in interprofessional teams is not new, but if nursing can eliminate incivility within its own ranks, we can model for others how intra and interprofessional teams can work collegially and effectively.

Cost cutting has always been an issue in healthcare, but we must become even more vigilant than in the past about giving away nursing duties to other, lower-paid disciplines or to non-RNs. We must restore our image as identifiable, professional, and trustworthy. To do so, we should be readily distinguishable from non RNs, unify, support one another, and maintain a high standard for ourselves and our colleagues.

In short, we must get our act together if we are to move forward. We do not want to be left behind, competing with each other over issues that should have been resolved years ago. Let's standardize orientations and residencies within similar healthcare organizations so we know that all new graduates get at least a minimum amount of instruction. Let's train our mentors and preceptors. Let's finally recognize that most patient care occurs in community settings and value what nurses do there. Let's encourage new and experienced nurses to explore new settings for nursing practice. Let's be sure not to lose the basics of patient care and comfort, even while we learn about and use cutting-edge technology.

Let's allow ourselves and each other to rest and restore our energies, and not look askance at a nurse who takes her vacation time or takes his lunch break or stays home when she's sick. Let's do away with the elitism that separates us from each other, prevents us from accomplishing everything we should, and prevents us from being able to present a unified image to the public. Let's make sure we are in the forefront of disaster and emergency preparedness by keeping abreast of what is happening in the world and of the potential for global issues to threaten healthcare in our nation and the safety of our patients.

KEY POINTS ABOUT THE FUTURE OF NURSING PRACTICE

Relationship with physicians

Bullying and incivility

Workload and burnout

Pay and poor working conditions

Back to basics

Elitism

Disunity

Public image

Ancillary staff

Care delivery

Insufficient jobs

Residencies, orientations, preceptors, and mentors

Communication and collaboration

Professionalism

Disaster preparation

References

American Nurses Association. (2014, May/June). Association news update; Welcome new specialty affiliates. *The American Nurse, 5.*

Baack, S., & Alfred, D. (2013). Nurses' preparedness and perceived competence in managing disasters. *Journal of Nursing Scholarship, 45*(3), 281–287.

Barnett, J. S., Minnick, A. F., & Norman, L. D. (2014). A description of U.S. post-graduation nurse residency programs. *Nursing Outlook, 62*(3), 174–184.

Budin, W. C., Brewer. C. S., Chao, Y. Y., & Kovner, C. (2013). Verbal abuse from nurse colleagues and work environment of early career registered nurses. *Journal f Nursing Scholarship, 45*(3), 308–316.

Castle, N. G. (2008). Special care units and their influence on nursing home occupancy characteristics. *Health Care Management Review, 33*(1), 79–91.

Iglehart, J. K. (2013). Expanding the role of advanced practice nurse practitioners: Risks and rewards. *The New England Journal of Medicine, 368*(20), 1,935–1,941.

Indiana State Nurses Association. (2014, February/March). Independent study: The evolving practice of nursing. *ISNA Bulletin, 7–10.*

Institute of Medicine. (2010). *Future of Nursing: Leading change, advancing health.* Retrieved from: http://www.iom.edu/Reports/2010/The-future-of-nursing-leading-change-advancing-health.aspx

Lavin, R. P. (2006). HIPAA and disaster research: Preparing to conduct research. *Disaster Management and Response, 4,* 32–36.

Lubbe, J. C., & Roets, L. (2014). Nurses' scope of practice and the implication for quality nursing care. *Journal of Nursing Scholarship, 46*(1), 58–64.

Neal-Boylan, L. (2012). *Nurses with disabilities: Professional issues and retention.* New York: Springer.

Neal-Boylan, L. (2013). *The nurse's reality gap: Overcoming barriers between academic achievement and clinical success.* Indianapolis, IN: Sigma Theta Tau Publishing.

Nightingale, F. (1860). *Notes on nursing: What it is and is not.* Retrieved from: http://digital.library.upenn.edu/women/nightingale/nursing/nursing.html#III

Rutherford, M. M. (2012). Nursing is the room rate. *Nursing Economics, 30*(4), 193–206.

Trossman, S. (2014, Jan/Feb). Toward civility: ANA, nurses promote strategies to prevent disruptive behaviors. *The American Nurse, 46*(1), 6.

Zhang, N. J., Unruh, L., & Wan, T. T. H. (2013). Gaps in nurse staffing and nursing home resident needs. *Nursing Economics, 31*(6), 289–297.

Chapter 9
Looking Toward the Future for Nursing Policy

"There is slush on the steps of the residence," said the nursing school matron, Essie. "Enter through the hospital, girls." Essie was always harsh and stern about not breaking "the rules," but protective all the same. She was seated in her nook at the entranceway of the nurses' residence as we returned from our weekend passes.

Essie started her day at 4 p.m. as house mother to us all and we knew her as the "no kissing in the reception room" lady. It was permissible, but not condoned, to bring a beau into the inner sanctum and hold hands. The reception room, with décor as old as the nursing school, was very large. This environment was more fitting for Miss Havisham receiving David Copperfield than it was for nursing students. We would enter in our starched, striped uniforms and white overskirts and starched white caps, polished white shoes and white nylons, just off duty at 4 p.m. on Sunday afternoon. An impatient boyfriend who had been carefully scrutinized by Essie was sitting awkwardly on a settee.

Boyfriends waited for that hour, before our dinner or evening tour of duty, to speak quietly of engagements, wedding plans, or a last goodbye before embarking to Korea and the war. Going out nearby with a beau to a movie was a treat and required permission. The scramble to find something to wear went from room to room. Gradually, as our friendships grew because of living and working together, we became aware of which friends had money.

The stipend from the hospital was $12 per month, and our labor was otherwise free in exchange for room and board and textbooks. I and a few others lived on that $12 per month. Since I was living at the nurses' residence, my mother figured that my needs were met.

One day, the director of the hospital was informed that an extraordinary event was to take place. The Duke and Duchess of Windsor were to visit and provide an endowment to the pediatric wing of the hospital. The director invited the royals to the residence for a reception following the ceremony. It was 1952, and as students, we did not question this bounty to our pediatric ward. At the time, I was president of our student council. The director of nurses requested that all students not on duty attend the reception, at which there would be tea poured from the hospital's silver tea service. As president of the student council, I was asked to pour the tea!

Probably one of the most significant influences on changes to modern nursing practice has been the Institute of Medicine (IOM) report issued in 2010. Together with the Robert Wood Johnson Foundation, they developed and released their report, "Future of Nursing: Leading Change, Advancing Health." There were four key initiatives:

- Nurses should practice to the full extent of their education and training.

- Nurses should achieve higher levels of education and training through an improved education system that promotes seamless academic progression.

- Nurses should be full partners, with physicians and other healthcare professionals, in redesigning healthcare in the United States.

- Effective workforce planning and policymaking require better data collection and an improved information infrastructure.

Tremendous effort is underway to improve nursing in all these areas. Organizations at the state and national levels have taken steps to comply with these initiatives and to make nurses aware of the need for change.

In early 2013, the American Nurses Association (ANA) launched its new 2-year strategic plan, citing five key points:

- Simplify the governance structure.

- Strengthen the constituent and state nurses' associations and ANA.

- Create and implement a high-growth membership organization.

- Develop a focused menu of programs, products, and services.

- Develop an integrated business and technology platform (ANA, 2014, p. 50).

In addition, the ANA promised to focus on eight "programmatic pillars" to prioritize their work:

- Leadership

- Cornerstone documents

- Scope of practice

- Care innovation

- Quality

- Work environment

- Safe staffing

- Healthy nurse (p. 50)

The ANA developed a leadership institute and resources to educate nurses about professional and other issues, recognized the scope and standards of specialties, and supports RNs and APRNs as they attempt to work to their fullest extent as recommended by the IOM. The national association has worked to influence national policy, advocate for and promote nursing quality and patient safety, advocate for a healthful work environment and the wellness of nurses, and explore ways to promote safe staffing (p. 52).

The National League for Nursing announced a commitment to four main areas for its 2013–2014 policy agenda:

- Access to quality healthcare for all

- Ethnic, cultural, and gender diversity

- Nurse workforce development

- The nurse faculty shortage (www.nln.org)

Between the two national nursing organizations, the mandates of the IOM are being taken seriously, and efforts to plan for the future are underway. I don't think it is unreasonable to wonder, though, if the ANA and the NLN were to merge into one organization, whether nurses wouldn't have more power to influence changes in healthcare and to enhance the public image of nurses. One organization such as this could also conceivably afford to keep membership prices low enough for any nurse, active or retired, to participate.

Along the same lines, we have two primary accrediting bodies for nursing education programs: the American Commission for Education in Nursing (ACEN, formerly the NLNAC) and the Commission on Collegiate Nursing Education (CCNE). Schools without graduate programs, particularly doctoral programs, typically start out with ACEN accreditation, but it is not uncommon for them to change to CCNE accreditation when they develop doctoral programs and to drop the ACEN. To remain in both is very costly to the college or university. Schools pay a great deal of money to have the required review and site visit, let alone to retain membership in each organization.

In addition, the NLN is a separate but sister organization to the ACEN, just as the American Association of Colleges of Nursing (AACN) is the parent organization of the CCNE. However, the AACN requires its own survey data from schools independent of those required by CCNE. A lot of duplication of effort takes place. These are but a few examples. This situation affects cost (which must be passed on to students in some form or fashion), workload for faculty and administrators, and most of all, the unity or disunity within the profession.

The Affordable Care Act (ACA)

The Affordable Care Act promises to bring significant changes to nursing practice. It is hoped that new models of care, such as patient-centered medical homes and increasing community-based care, will result in savings in healthcare. However, advanced practice nurses are needed to fill the gap in primary care and to expand the scope of practice. States are considering legislation to accept the Advanced Practice Nurse Model Act to allow independent practice for nurse practitioners (Fairman, Rowe, Hassmiller, & Shalala, 2011). While the nursing shortage has been somewhat reduced because economic necessity has driven some retired nurses back to work, many areas still lack APRNs (Iglehart, 2013), and many nurse practitioners are choosing to specialize instead of entering or remaining in primary care (Iglehart, 2013).

As of 2013, the United States boasted of 3.1 million licensed registered nurses. Projections continue to be optimistic that the profession will remain among the most desirable occupations for the foreseeable future. The demand will continue to grow as aging nurses retire. The Nursing Workforce Development programs, in use since 1964 under Title VIII of the Public Health Service Act, continue to support nursing education and solutions to the nursing shortage (http://www.aacn.nche.edu/government-affairs/TitleVIII.pdf) ("Nursing workforce," 2013).

Not only does the ACA improve access to care and reimbursement to APRNs, it also enhances preventive care services and provides funding for nursing education and nurse-managed/led centers. The legislation supports grants for nursing education, workforce diversity, and nurse retention. It also supports nursing specialties and nurses who pursue advanced education (ANA, 2012; Wakefield, 2010).

Mental Health Care

According to the ACA, mental-health and substance-abuse treatment are essential health benefits. Consequently, health-insurance plans, regardless of type, must cover the care of people with mental-health disorders. There are not enough mental-health providers to serve these patients, however. (http://www.healthaffairs.org/healthpolicybriefs/brief.php?brief_id=112) ("Health Policy Brief," 2014). While nursing students typically receive education in psychiatric issues, they will likely need more varied and in-depth training and experience with populations of patients who have mental-health disorders or substance-abuse problems. In addition, it is important that the profession encourage students returning to school to obtain the APRN to consider the field of psychiatric nursing.

Prevention and Population-Based Care

In the future, there will be more emphasis on disease prevention and wellness, although nurses have carried that banner throughout their history. The healthcare world has recognized that it is less expensive to support preventive measures than to care for people after they become ill or disabled.

Nurses will also be more involved in population-based care, and will need a working knowledge of epidemiology. While many treatments will be developed for the individual due to the advances in genetics and the human genome, much of healthcare delivery will be based on care of populations with similar healthcare issues.

The role of nurse navigator will take on importance as patients continue to require experts to help guide them through the maze of healthcare options and providers. Other nurse roles new to the profession are likely to appear.

The Nursing Workforce

Review and analysis of the nursing workforce is a key strategy as the profession plans for the future. In 2003, Bleich et al. conducted an integrative review of reports from formal documents, articles, and consultants. They concluded that the workforce shortage was a complex problem that could be divided into national and institutional themes. National themes included healthcare economics, inadequate workforce planning, workforce development, and concern for the public's health (p. 71). Institutional themes included supply of nurses, demand for services, work environment, and leadership (p. 71). Interestingly, and not surprisingly, the institutional themes have been prevalent throughout this book and remain areas of concern for nurses today.

Bleich et al. found that national, institutional, and individual imperatives emerged from their research. The national imperatives included the need to develop public policies "favoring fair reimbursement for basic and advanced nursing services" (p. 73) and the need to allocate some federal monies to planning and developing the healthcare workforce.

Improving the work climate (including safety and salary adjustments), the integration of technology, academic and service partnerships, and leadership development were the institutional imperatives. The researchers challenged nurses to develop a voice in policy and professional decisions and to "recognize that the profession of nursing will continue to change" (p. 74).

We continue to need and collect workforce data. The Robert Wood Johnson Foundation funded briefs to provide guidance that states can use to build systems to collect and maintain data (National League for Nursing, 2014). The briefs explain the need to collect data and develop better systems for doing so, provide suggestions for developing and maintaining a system, and describe some successful approaches for data collection.

The Nursing Workforce Development programs fall under Title VIII of the Public Health Service Act (42 U. S. C. 296 *et seq.*). These have helped increase the supply of nurses since 1964. The programs help fund nursing student education and promote the education of nurse practitioners to work in primary care, nurses who choose to work in rural and underserved areas, and the preparation of nursing faculty.

Another more recent study (ANA, 2014) found that lower nurse-patient ratios and higher numbers of bachelor's degrees resulted in fewer deaths among surgical patients. The study was "the largest and most detailed analysis to date of patient outcomes associated with nurse staff education in Europe" (p. 7). Linda Aiken, one of the researchers, stated that the European study results were comparable to findings in the United States (ANA, 2014).

Much of my research in recent years has focused on RNs with physical and/or sensory disabilities (Neal-Boylan, 2012). It is clear that these nurses suffer discrimination in the workplace, despite the Americans with Disabilities Act Amendment of 2008 (ADAAA). These nurses have a tendency to leave their jobs and, sometimes, the profession because others fear they will jeopardize patient safety. This is another example of our inability to harness the strength we have in the more than 3,100,000 nurses in this country. If we make all RNs feel valued and feel that there is a place for them in the profession, there need be no nursing shortage, nor difficulty strengthening our workforce and the influence nurses have in society and on policy.

The workforce has been affected by nurses who might previously have retired, but who have remained in the workforce. Auerbach, Buerhaus, and Staiger (2014) reported:

> The recession, and its lingering effects, may have temporarily delayed the retirement of older RNs because of income security reasons. However, we found there has been a large shift toward later retirements during the past four decades that was independent of any effects associated with the economic downturns that occurred in this period. Baby-boomer RNs will eventually retire. Nonetheless, this shift has lasting implications for workforce projections, hospitals and other settings that employ older RNs in particular, and policy makers are concerned with ensuring an adequate RN supply and protecting the quality and safety of patient care in the United States. (http://content.healthaffairs.org/content/early/2014/07/10/hlthaff.2014.0128.early)

The researchers went on to say that as nurses age, they move out of hospitals and are more likely to work in community settings. They suggest that this could be an advantage in light of the ACA because more nurses will be needed to perform tasks associated with the transition and coordination of care.

Nurse-managed health clinics (Title III of the Public Service Act) help support training of the future primary-care workforce by serving as clinical sites for healthcare-provider students and new graduates. APRNs manage the clinics, but an interprofessional team provides care to underserved individuals (www.nncc.us/site/).

Commitment to Veterans

The AACN has developed the Joining Forces initiative and has partnered with the Jonas Center for Nursing and Veterans Health care to support veterans in nursing schools and in practice. The Health Resources Services Administration (HRSA) has provided funding support for schools of nursing and other health professions that work toward establishing course and credit equivalencies for military experience. It is important that schools of nursing determine how much, if at all, military experience and training weigh toward nursing education. Schools and healthcare professional programs will soon be competing to attract the large number of veterans seeking to return to school.

Diversity

With encouragement from the Institute of Medicine, funding sources, and national nursing organizations such as the AACN, the profession continues to promote a diverse workforce. The AACN notes that there is an upward trend in minority group participation in baccalaureate and graduate programs over the last 10 years. However, students are overwhelmingly White in each of these programs. The AACN also notes that males comprise 11% of the nurse workforce, as opposed to 9% in 2004. The AACN has collaborated with others to obtain support for increasing students from diverse backgrounds in nursing schools (http://www.aacn.nche.edu/government-affairs/Student-Diversity-FS.pdf).

People with disabilities are also a diverse group who are often overlooked and underserved. It is time that nursing organizations looked at how we might revise or eliminate the technical standards we use to admit students to school and the archaic job descriptions we rely on to determine whether a nurse is competent to work. Let's work together to define the "essential functions" of nursing work. Again, if our focus is on critical thinking and judgment, why can't we admit bright, otherwise capable students who may need to compensate by using technology or other assistance to become nurses? Why do we continue to push nurses with disabilities out of nursing when our fears are unfounded?

Home Care

Job growth for nurses in hospitals is expected to slow while outpatient, community, and long-term settings are likely to see a rise. Hospitals are being asked to reduce costs and inefficiencies (Cipriano, 2014). While perhaps home, community, and public health are finally being recognized by the profession as areas that deserve more didactic and clinical time to prepare nurses to care for patients, the majority of whom reside in our communities, there are still limits on APRN practice in these settings. The Home Health Care Planning Improvement Act (H.R. 2504, S. 1332) would allow APRNs to certify Medicare patients to receive skilled care in the home. The bill has been defeated in the past but is currently under review again.

I started in home care many years ago as a case manager and later worked as a rehabilitation clinical nurse specialist. Home care is very different from inpatient care, but nurses often assume that it requires less skill or ability. Quite the contrary. Nurses working in home care must be very confident and competent because they are largely autonomous (Neal, 1999) and rarely have access to high-tech equipment or other people in the home setting. Home care requires the nurse to be adaptable, flexible, and highly skilled. Nurses must be comfortable working in unstructured settings.

We thought that home healthcare would gain increased recognition from nurses and the public with the advent of the Prospective Payment System legislation in the 1990s. However, it has remained somewhat of a stepchild—a last resort for nurses who no longer want or feel they are able to work in the hospital, a flexible option for nurses with young children, and a refuge for nurses whose hearts lie with community health. Today, more new graduates are testing the home care waters because it is more difficult to get a job in the hospital right out of school. However, it is necessary for new graduates—and experienced inpatient nurses, for that matter—to get a long and comprehensive orientation to home healthcare because it is so different from the hospital.

I have always thought of home care as a well-kept secret, although not for lack of trying by home health nurses, the *Home Healthcare Nurse* journal, and the National Association for Home Care & Hospice. Thankfully, there is a new international organization of home health nurses, the International Home Care Nurses Organization, that is beginning to gain traction.

Home healthcare is a perfect venue for APRNs. They can conduct holistic assessments and, if eventually allowed, write orders for care that will consider the patient's lifestyle and financial barriers. Physicians don't seem to enjoy writing and keeping up with orders for home care patients and are often "shooting in the dark" because they are unable to see their patients for extended periods of time. In contrast, the APRN could see the patient in the home as often as needed and justified by Medicare or insurance. The Home Health Care Planning Improvement Act would allow APRNs and clinical nurse specialists to certify home health services. Its passage is clearly in alignment with the goals of the IOM report (www.aacn.nche.edu).

APRN Consensus Model and Removal of Practice Barriers

APRNs practice as nurse practitioners, nurse midwives, clinical nurse specialists, and nurse anesthetists. The profession has worked hard to develop the Consensus Model for APRN Regulation so that a uniform title and standard regulations would safeguard practice and allow these nurses to move seamlessly throughout the United States. The model is scheduled for implementation in 2015. Nurses in any of these roles, and certified to practice, will use the title APRN, will hold both an RN and APRN license, will be able to practice independently from physicians, and will have full prescriptive authority (Cahill, Alexander, & Gross, 2014).

The Consensus Model will eliminate a significant barrier to the practice of nurse practitioners by standardizing the scope of practice within the United States. This is particularly important in light of the ACA and its intent to use NPs more frequently and fully in primary care (Gutchell, Idzik, & Lazear, 2014). Fairman et al. (2011) argued that "the critical factors limiting nurse practitioners' capacity to practice to the full extent of their education, training, and competence are state-based regulatory barriers" (p. 194).

Globalization of Healthcare

Healthcare is becoming increasingly international. Nurses move across international borders to provide care and influence health practices and policies. Nurses may be educated in one country and work in another.

According to Jones and Sherwood (2014), there are four major reasons globalization is important to nursing:

- Ubiquitous nursing shortages
- The aging nurse workforce
- Changes occurring in health systems to contain cost and efficiently deliver quality care
- The call to meet the needs of the world population

Jones and Sherwood note:

> To evaluate these global issues as well as new and emerging workforce models will require information gathering based on an agreed-upon core set of common data elements about where domestically educated nurses and IENs [internationally educated nurses] practice, their roles and functions, and if and how they move over time. (p. 62)

There will likely be increased emphasis on communicable and infectious diseases worldwide as people continue to travel widely. Nurses will need to be knowledgeable about illnesses they have not previously had to consider.

Technology and Informatics

The use of technology in healthcare has been a common topic of discussion and debate in recent years, particularly with the advent of the ACA (Clancy et al., 2014). A recent study revealed that nurses are very supportive of the standardization of technology goods and services to deliver high-quality care (Burnes, Bolton, Gassert, & Cipriano, 2008). However, nurses continue to have difficulty using electronic health records to research or report data (Clancy et al., 2014).

Most likely, technology will become more prevalent in healthcare planning and delivery. For nurses, this means being knowledgeable and comfortable with its use or being replaced by others who are. Schools of nursing are beginning to incorporate classes in informatics and the use of electronic health records into curricula.

High-fidelity mannequins have been in use for quite a while now. Like any technology, they are sometimes overused out of necessity or convenience, depending on the perspective. In either case, they have become a mainstay in schools that can afford them and have offered a remedy, in part, to the difficulty in locating sufficient clinical placements for students. Also, when used intelligently, they can prepare students for not only the clinical components of care delivery, but also the unique types of communication and decision-making that occur in healthcare organizations. Nonetheless, some survey respondents said that this type of simulation equipment is overused and is not the "be-all and end-all" to preparing new graduates for the real world.

As we become more comfortable using new technology, it is vital that nurses not lose sight of the importance of the basics of nursing care. This was clearly articulated by many survey respondents, and I agree. When we surrender morning care to others, for example, we lose the opportunity to build a rapport with the patient, conduct a head-to-toe assessment, and provide truly holistic care. In many settings, it has become so difficult to find time to be present for patients and families, yet this is what patients and families value most about nurses. They trust us above others because they expect that we will listen, interpret, and guide without the interference of an agenda. We are theirs. If we turn over that quality of nursing, we risk losing our identity. After all, any good health professional can be caring, observe monitors, and adjust IVs. We are known for demonstrating care and comfort, and for being the liaison between the frightening world of illness and the chance for pain relief, quality of life, or a dignified death.

Futures Thinking

Nurses are hearing more about futures studies and futures thinking. According to Foresight Education and Research Network (FERN; 2010), those who study the future concern themselves with futures that might occur, that are very likely to occur, and preferred futures. "Futures strategizing offers the means to counter negativism through the creation of positive and desirable futures" (Freed & McLaughlin, 2011, p. 175). According to Freed and McLaughlin, nurse educators should think like futurists to inculcate futures thinking into their students. They advise that the following strategies be incorporated into nursing education: forecasting, strategic foresight, backcasting, rearview-mirror analysis, and the futures wheel (p. 176–177).

Genomics

Genomics is an area that continues to grow and apply to healthcare delivery. Nurses must be educated to interpret this research to application. Genomic research has implications for diagnoses and treatment, and nurses need to be able to educate patients and evaluate new ideas and projects. Genomics will affect nursing education, research, clinical care, public health, ethics, and leadership, and nurses should be prepared to meet these challenges (Conley et al., 2013; Jenkins & Calzone, 2012).

Daack-Hirsch, Dieter, and Quinn Griffin (2011) proposed suggestions for incorporating genomic concepts into undergraduate education. They recommended using genomics as a thread throughout the curriculum, developing required or elective courses, and offering clinical experiences as options for integrating the material. Williams et al. (2011) described successful strategies that nursing faculty can use to increase their own expertise in genomics so they are confident in developing curricula for their students.

Leadership

Throughout the book, we have quoted nurses who made mention of the need for unified leadership and leaders who understand the issues facing clinical nurses. Many surveyed nurses expressed interest in participating in policy making, lobbying, and decision-making that would affect the entire profession. Many nurses—particularly those who cannot afford the time or money to participate in professional associations—do not know how to parlay their interest into action. They want and need leaders who will reach out to them.

The issue of unity is relevant to this discussion because, as has been mentioned, organizations are fragmented, and this prevents nurses from speaking with one voice. Nursing associations and journals compete with each other for membership, yet many of their causes are the same.

Nurses working at the bedside, unless they are in school, may perceive themselves as far away from the ivory tower, without the means to convey their views of proposed solutions to those who publish and attend national meetings. Older nurses in particular may have a lot to say, especially when they are able to speak to the changes that have faced nursing over time. I don't think we are harnessing their power, nor that of retired nurses, who often continue nursing activities, and this influences public perception (Neal-Boylan, Cocca, & Carnoali, 2009).

Conclusion

Several issues related to healthcare policy have the potential to affect nursing, and more arise every day. Many nurse executives and educators are aware of these issues because they are in positions that require them to advocate for or argue against them or to educate students. However, I submit that many nurses at every level of education and position are unaware of the most pressing policy issues of the day and how they affect nurses.

Clearly, 3,100,000 nurses present a potentially powerful voice if all are knowledgeable about the issues, are unified, and are willing to work and speak together as a profession. As the profession prepares for the future and nursing roles change to accommodate a very different healthcare landscape, it is important that we eliminate our divisiveness and competition with one another, close ranks, and finally achieve many of the goals that have eluded us.

KEY POINTS ABOUT THE FUTURE OF NURSING AND HEALTH POLICY

Affordable Care Act

Mental health care

Prevention and population-based care

Nursing workforce

Commitment to veterans

Diversity

Home care

APRN Consensus Model

Globalization of healthcare

Technology and informatics

Futures thinking

Genomics

Leadership

References

ANA. (2012, June 29). The Supreme Court decision matters for registered nurses, their families and their patients. *American Nurses Association,* 1–3. Retrieved from www.nursingworld.org/healthcarereform

ANA. (2014, March/April). Better nurse staffing, education lead to better outcomes. *The American Nurse, 7.*

ANA. (2014). Issues up close: ANA: Moving forward-mission possible. *American Nurse Today, (8)*1, 50–52.

Auerbach, D. I., Buerhaus, P. I., & Staiger, D. O. (2014 July). Registered nurses are delaying retirement, a shift that has contributed to recent growth in the nurse workforce. *Health Affairs.* DOI: 10.1377/hlthaff.2014.0128.

Bleich, M. R., Hewlett, P. O., Santos, R., Rice, R. B., Cox, K. S., & Richmeier, S. (2003). Analysis of the nursing workforce crisis: A call to action. *The American Journal of Nursing, 103*(4), 66–74.

Burnes Bolton, L., Gassert, C. A., & Cipriano, P. (2008). Smart technology, enduring solutions: Technology solutions can make care safer and more efficient. *Journal of Healthcare Information Management, 22*(4), 24–30.

Cahill, M., Alexander, M., & Gross, L. (2014). The 2014 NCSBN consensus report on APRN regulation. *Journal of Nursing Regulation, 4*(4), 5–12.

Cipriano, P. F. (2014). The disappearing inpatient. *American Nurse Today, 9*(1), 6.

Clancy, T. R., Bowles, K. H., Gelinas, L., Androwich, I., Delaney, C., Matney, S., … Westra, B. (2014). A call to action: Engage in big data science. *Nursing Outlook, 62*(1), 64–65.

Conley, Y. P., Biesecker, L. G., Gonsalves, S., Merkel, C. J., Kirk, M., Aouizerat, B. E. (2013). Current and emerging technology approaches in genomics. *Journal of Nursing Scholarship, 45*(19), 5–14.

Daack-Hirsch, S., Dieter, C., & Quinn Griffin, M. T. (2011). Integrating genomics into undergraduate nursing education. *Journal of Nursing Scholarship, 43*(3), 223–230.

Fairman, J. A., Rowe, J. W., Hassmiller, S., & Shalala, D. E. (2011). Broadening the scope of nursing practice. *The New England Journal of Medicine, 364*(3), 193–196.

Foresight Education and Research Network (FERN). (2010). Glossary. Retrieved from www.fernweb.org/page/Glossary

Freed, P. E., & McLaughlin, D. E. (2011). Futures thinking: Preparing nurses to think for tomorrow. *Nursing Education Perspectives, 32*(3), 173–178.

Gutchell, V., Idzik, S., & Lazear, J. (2014). An evidence-based path to removing APRN practice barriers. *The Journal for Nurse Practitioners, 10*(4), 255–261.

Health policy brief: Mental health parity. (2014). *Health Affairs*. Retrieved from http://www.healthaffairs.org/healthpolicybriefs/brief.php?brief_id=112

Home Health Care Planning Improvement Act of 2013, H.R. 2504, S. 1332.

Iglehart, J. K. (2013). Expanding the role of advanced nurse practitioners—risks and rewards. *New England Journal of Medicine, 368*:1,935–1,941.

Institute of Medicine. (2010). The future of nursing: Leading change, advancing health. Washington, DC: National Academies Press.

Jenkins, J. F., & Calzone, K. A. (2012). Are nursing faculty ready to integrate genomic content into curricula? *Nurse Education, 37*(1), 25–29.

Jones, C. B., & Sherwood, G. D. (2014). The globalization of the nursing workforce: Pulling the pieces together. *Nursing Outlook, 62, 59–63.*

National League for Nursing. (2014). Issue briefs discuss the need for nursing workforce data. *Nursing Education Policy Newsletter, 11*(2), 1.

National Nursing Centers Consortium: Keeping our nation healthy. (2014). Retrieved from www.nncc.us/site/

Neal, L. J. (1999). Validating and refining the Neal theory of home health nursing practice. *Home Health Care Management & Practice, 12*(2), 16–25.

Neal-Boylan, L. (2012). *Nurses with disabilities: Professional issues and retention.* New York: Springer.

Neal-Boylan, L. J., Cocca, K., & Carnoali, B. (2009). The benefits to working for retired nurses. *Geriatric Nursing, 30*(6), 378–383.

Nursing workforce development programs. (2013). Retrieved from http://www.aacn.nche.edu/government-affairs/TitleVIII.pdf

Policy brief: The changing landscape: Nursing student diversity on the rise. Retrieved from http://www.aacn.nche.edu/government- affairs/Student-Diversity-FS.pdf

Public Health Service Act of 1964, 42 U. S. C. 296 et seq.

Wakefield, M. K. (2010). Nurses and the Affordable Care Act. *American Journal of Nursing, 110*(9), 11.

Williams, J. K., Prows, C. A., Conley, Y. P., Eggert, J., Kirk, M., & Nichols, F. (2011). Strategies to prepare faculty to integrate genomics into nursing education programs. *Journal of Nursing Scholarship, 43*(3), 231–238.

Chapter 10
Conclusions

Two or three months to go—our last year as students coming
to a close. The hospital, disregarding what today would be
considered "unfair labor practices," assigned us "in-charge"
status on the private floors. The evening shift, from 4 p.m.
to 12 midnight, was usually quiet, the instructors assured us.
There were black velvet bands on our student caps. They gave
us status. We were almost finished, all knowing. It never occurred to us that being unlicensed, we were liable.

We were rather impressed with our patients: wealthy and
demanding, with real silver tea and coffee services brought to
their bedsides, food that was exceptionally fine for hospital
fare, physicians who were, in their time, renowned in their
specialties and somewhat subservient to their patients. Beautiful lingerie and slippers and the occasional high-heeled mules
were their bedclothes. We marveled—especially those like me,
who lived on the $12 per month stipend granted by the hos-
pital. Otherwise, our nursing services were free. I prospered,
though. Fran Levy did have money. Her father, a pharmacist
in Schenectady, sent it to her, and she shopped—a sweater for
her and one for me. With $6, I bought a short-sleeved wool
sweater and, after borrowing a bag or gloves and a coat from
Donna, I managed.

The best time to be on shift was at 11:30 in the evening. The halls were dark and quiet. One could hear the shoes of the evening supervisor as she made her rounds and walked to the desk, crisp and efficient and single (we presumed), to get the evening report. Shortly after that, the night shift came on, and we gave them report and left the floor. Our evening wasn't over, however. It had just begun. We all appeared in the basement dining room to have "lunch" with the interns and residents. The general flirting led to several marriages after graduation.

I still remember Sunday evening chicken and superb coffee ice cream, returning to the residence for bed, and getting up for class at 7 a.m. Young and healthy, we thought it all great fun and very glamorous. As students, we were all very close and caring, and in and out of each other's rooms constantly. Advice about boyfriends, makeup, clothes, and smoking was continuous.

Being in charge of a floor meant, of course, that you could not leave your post until relieved by the next shift. This became a deprivation one Sunday afternoon at about 5 p.m. The kitchen staff brought up the trays, and with them the most exciting news: Marilyn Monroe was on the 11th floor (the most elite floor of all), visiting her mother-in-law, Mrs. Miller! But I remained at my post.

The purpose of this book has been to remind nurses that we have been revisiting many of the same issues since the early days of the profession. I thought that if we could see that many nursing issues, while somewhat morphed over the years, have continued to plague us, we might be more inclined to resolve them once and for all. Several themes have emerged as thus far unresolved or inadequately so.

Elitism

Since 1893, when the Association of Superintendents of Training Schools was formed, there has been divisiveness among nurses regarding decisions made without the input of bedside nurses. Lavinia Dock (as cited in

Birnbach & Lewenson, 1991) asked us to avoid clique-like behavior in 1896. It is rare today to have a well-known and influential nurse leader who is current clinically to the point of understanding the issues faced by nurses at the bedside. My academic and researcher colleagues will say that it is nearly impossible to teach classes, conduct high-quality research, publish, serve on committees and boards, *and* maintain a clinical practice. By the same token, nurses who primarily work clinically should be comfortable reading and critically analyzing research, employing evidence-based practice, and generally using a scientific attitude in their work.

I see two solutions to this problem, although I am certain others would have additional suggestions:

- Nurse leaders who serve in decision-making positions that affect the profession as a whole must interact with patients in direct care roles on a *per diem* basis, even if it is once a month or during the summer. This should be true of nursing faculty, as well. I don't see how one can teach students about current practice without engaging in it oneself. Besides, bedside nurses and students are more likely to respect nurse educators and leaders who can "walk the walk." Leaders of specialty nursing organizations should be chosen in part based on their current understanding of the clinical issues facing that specialty.

- There should be a targeted effort to include nurses who provide direct care on a full-time basis in high-level meetings that require decisions that affect the profession. They and their input should be recruited and valued. Todays' technology should allow full participation without an excess commitment of time and energy.

Disunity

Elitism and disunity are kissing cousins. Disunity affects so much of what we have tried to accomplish as a profession. We have failed to effectively harness the power of 3,100,000 nurses because our organizations and relationships are fragmented. This has influenced our approach to policy, relationships with physicians, and recognition by other healthcare providers and the public. Isabel Hampton Robb (as cited in Birnbach & Lewenson, 1991) exhorted us to draw closer together as a profession because "we know that nurses are *made* not born" (p. 100).

Early on, the best students in nurse training schools were tracked into leadership roles, while their classmates became private duty nurses. Although what we do today is less blatant, we do give our baccalaureate graduates the impression that it is vital and necessary for them to go back to graduate school as soon as possible after graduation.

Many schools now have programs that move students directly from baccalaureate classes into masters or doctoral programs. Not only does this instill the idea that staying at the bedside an associate-degree or a baccalaureate-prepared nurse is somehow inadequate, but these direct-entry programs channel students into careers in nursing before they have a true understanding of what nursing is or what nurses do. They are pigeonholed into a career, usually as a nurse practitioner, before they know how to be a nurse. We want them to think like nurses—after all, this is what distinguishes nurse practitioners from physician's assistants—but they don't have time to assimilate as nurses before they take on the weighty responsibility and liability of being an APRN. Besides, there are so many things one can do as a nurse, they need time to explore their options and see what will really suit them. No less important for the profession is the fact that we need the young and strong at the hospital bedside doing the physical work required of taking care of the very ill because older nurses are less able to perform that kind of heavy work.

We must discourage multiple specialty organizations and encourage full participation in our national organization, the American Nurses Association (ANA), with membership fees that are affordable and realistic. It is important that the ANA advocate for policy based on member input, not focus on politics or supporting politicians or political parties. We must make professional conferences affordable and make all nurses feel welcome by lowering registration costs, forgoing high-priced hotels (perhaps in favor of hosting universities), and including topics that can be directly applied to improving patient care and the work life of nurses. There should be fewer journals, and they should be affordable and comprehensible to all nurses.

If nurses learn to critically analyze research while in the undergraduate program, they will be prepared to read scholarly journals. Instead, we have a spectrum of journals that require the reader to have a PhD to understand and journals that only nurses involved in direct patient care can appreciate.

Not Everyone Can Be a Nurse

Early in the 20th century, nurses worked hard to develop rigorous admission criteria. It was important to them that it be understood that not everyone can be a nurse. Additionally, early nurse leaders recognized the need to admit only those students who could think critically. We have reached a point where we accept students who may (or may not) have the right academic credentials but who are clearly not suited to perform nursing work. Many arrive with misconceptions—thinking they will become nurse practitioners, for example. They scarcely recognize that they must learn how to be nurses first, and that there is far more to being an NP than writing prescriptions. Additionally, it is becoming increasingly common to see students who cannot cope with college life, let alone be considered emotionally strong enough to support patients in their time of need.

We should be more careful about whom we admit. It may be unwieldy to interview several hundred undergraduate students, but are there other ways, such as a required essay written under close supervision, to find out more about how a prospective student thinks. Essays that require problem-solving skills might enable us to assess if the prospective student already knows how to think critically. Increased use of group interviews might allow us to see who is inquisitive, who is a leader, and how each candidate interacts with others. We must encourage students to question and require them to compare and contrast sources of information, defend their decisions, and carefully analyze potential solutions to patient problems. Students often think there is only one answer, and they want their professors to simply provide that answer. The care of individuals is inherently individualized, however. Nursing students should be required to propose more than one possible solution, treatment, therapy, etc., instead of using cookie-cutter approaches.

Broad Base of Knowledge

It is not enough for students to receive a liberal educational foundation. They must be inquisitive and read and write well. Early nurse leaders lamented that even native-born nursing students couldn't speak or write English well (Snively, as cited in Birnbach & Lewenson, 1991), and that knowledge of English and literature were necessary. They required students to be "independent searchers of knowledge" (Gillette, as cited in Birnbach & Lewenson, 1991, p. 37) and to seek out information rather than expecting it to be provided to them.

Professionals can speak intelligently about what's happening in the world and about a variety of topics. Much of this comes from being well-read, as does good writing. One's vocabulary and sentence structure are often influenced by reading a wide variety of good literature. We are challenged by technology and the increasing tendency to use sound bites and tweets to convey messages. Allowing nursing students to bypass the requirements to write and speak well and read widely will continue to keep us mired in the pool shared by technicians and unskilled workers.

Clinical Experience

The profession recognized early on that the clinical experiences with which students were provided were key to their development as nurses. The questions of how much is enough and appropriate use of clinical time still exist, however. Students often ran the hospital. While that is clearly too much responsibility, I think they need more than they usually have. We have been saying for years that students need to manage a typical load of patients before graduating instead of just one or two patients. We should make this happen.

Students need more exposure to healthcare organizations and the formal and informal structures of these organizations. The ability to provide clinical care is the priority, but to survive as new graduates, they must also know how to prevent being bullied, how to be a good team member, whom to go to for what, and how to speak and interact effectively with colleagues.

The nurse residency is not a new idea, but is finally gaining traction. We will never think we have enough clinical time, but we can make the time students *do* have in clinical replicate the real world as much as possible. Simulation can only go so far. It cannot prepare students for the unexpected. Moreover, humans are full of surprises, especially when ill. Is it time to extend baccalaureate education by one year to accommodate all that the modern nurse needs to know?

With the increased emphasis on prevention, population-based care, and community health, it is important that students have more realistic and more frequent experiences in public health and home health. Too often, clinical hours in these areas are sacrificed to give students time in the hospital, even though most actual patient care occurs in community settings. In the early days of the profession, public and community health were valued, and a large part of the nursing role involved teaching how to prevent illness. Nurses who worked in public health were the elite. Hospitals were not nice places to be. (They still aren't, although for different reasons.) Patients continue to be exposed to iatrogenic infections and antibiotic-resistant infections. Today, hospitals are places for the very ill or for post-surgical patients. This has been an insurance-driven phenomenon but given the exposure to infection, the expense of hospital care, and the inconsistency in providers, it is better in many cases for patients to be cared for at home. We must model for students that nursing care provided in community settings is respected, valued, and necessary.

After 9/11, there was a tremendous focus on preparing healthcare personnel to participate in disaster planning. This urgency reappears whenever there is a concern about bioterrorism. However, I think we have diminished our emphasis on disaster planning and emergency preparedness. During wartime in the 1940s, nurses took action to propose postgraduate education and refresher courses for nurses to prepare them for war and emergencies that might arise. It might behoove us to consider increasing our emphasis in a coordinated manner to ensure that nursing students receive standardized disaster training and that nurses are provided with opportunities to learn or be refreshed on this material.

Relationships

Our relationships with physician colleagues have clearly improved, although isolated cases still occur in which nurses are treated without respect. We can only hope that new generations of physicians are being taught to be more collegial and interprofessional. That seems to be the case. The more responsibility we gain, however, the more threatening we become, even when physicians are unable to continue to manage all that is expected of them. I think they are in crisis. They are losing their hold on primary care, they are no longer guaranteed wealth, and they are no longer, as a group, held in high esteem, above all other mortals. They will need to come to grips with these changes, and we can help them. We can continue to teach them that we are colleagues and that one does not become a nurse because one can't get into medical school. The more professional we are and appear, the less likely they will be to treat us as subservient.

Diploma nursing schools were often very strict and motivated students with threats and punishments. Today, we are facing incivility, most frequently between experienced nurses and new graduates. In many nursing schools, we have gone from being benevolent dictators to being nurturers who feel it is our obligation to make students happy and contented. While we must be fair to all, we do our students a disservice by not preparing them for the real world in which employees and employers expect everyone to pull their weight and not complain about it.

In the early days, when nurses graduated, they became part of a club of sorts. *Esprit de corps* helped support new nurses and instilled pride in the profession. The differences between then and now are that new graduates were taught to respect their elders and the nurses with experience, accept that there was an awful lot still to be learned, and be willing to learn from others and to seek out information themselves.

In 1930, Wheeler lamented that we were admitting unqualified students who had "personality difficulties" (p. 189). They were overbearing and unkind. They lacked intelligence and organizational skills, were unable to "solve problems [and] make judgments" (Urch, as cited in Birnbach & Lewenson, 1991, p. 234). I often hear from faculty (and have myself experienced) that students are sometimes rude, disruptive, and overbearing. We have not had much success, it would appear, in making sure we admit students who are respectful, diligent, and appreciative of the privilege of becoming nurses. However, we can make them what we want them to be and increase our expectations for professional behavior. We can also heap praise upon the students who do show appropriate deference and a sincere desire to learn.

I think a component of incivility is that nurses are very tired. They are tired of trying to do more with less; of working overtime; of rarely taking their earned breaks and vacations; of dealing with rude patients, students, doctors, and administrators; and of not being valued commensurate with their knowledge and ability. I don't think 12-hour days have helped us. Many nurses like 12-hour days because they have 4 days off each week, but realistically, how effective can one be in those last few hours? Nurses in the 1920s picketed for 8-hour workdays because they knew even then that 12-hour shifts were too much. Nightingale (1860) and later Wolf (as cited in Birnbach & Lewenson, 1991) said that nurses need their rest and need to feel that they are developing intellectually to gain satisfaction from their work.

Public Image

Eliminating a standard nursing uniform was a mistake. We thought doing so would make us appear more professional, but it has succeeded in accomplishing the opposite. No one knows who we are, little girls and boys do not have a vision of the nurse in their heads to motivate them to want to be that person, and others have moved into the breach to pick up many of our former duties and responsibilities.

Public image goes well beyond the uniform. Nurses with heavy makeup, fancy manicures, tattoos, dangling earrings, and an unkempt appearance make us all look unprofessional and uneducated. It is not that I am being old-fashioned. The simple fact is that for the present, people still expect professionals to dress, look, and behave conservatively. It is difficult to have confidence in someone who looks like they don't have confidence in themselves.

Ancillary Staff

We seem to have a love/hate relationship with ancillary staff. We love having help, but we must remain constantly vigilant of unlicensed personnel who take on nursing work. We have given over much to licensed practical nurses, students, and nurse's aides. In doing so, we have diluted our roles and have contributed to the difficulty distinguishing who is the nurse. The public calls anyone in scrubs a nurse. We must correct them, more clearly define our territory for the public, and establish how we see the use of ancillary personnel.

I am hardly the first to suggest that associate-degree nurses could be used in future to support the baccalaureate-prepared nurse. The associate-degree program was originally intended to train nursing technicians, not nursing professionals. Associate-degree nurses have a broad liberal education but typically lack knowledge and skills in leadership, theory, and research. Ideally, only the baccalaureate nurse and the nurse's aide should remain, and the roles of LPN- and ADN-prepared nurse be eliminated. This is unlikely to happen, however, since many have called for this change for countless years without success.

In 1970, Alfano asked if "registered professional nurses" were necessary because we had delegated so much care to ancillary personnel.

She asked us to reevaluate who we were and our functions. "We are so busy identifying our roles that we can't hear the voices calling for those basic comforts that were once the very reason of our existence" (p. 2,116). So many surveyed nurses asked that we get back to basics and remember that the basics of nursing care are what the patients truly value about nursing. We must not lose ground we have gained in taking on some of the tasks that used to be the purview of the physician. But, let's not lose the basics of care and comfort as we do so.

Diversity

As a profession, we seem to recognize more than ever that we lack sufficient diversity to represent the general population of patients for whom we care. Thankfully, there are more men in nursing now, but we must strengthen our efforts to recruit students and nurses of diverse backgrounds and to welcome them into the profession. I include not only people of color and varying ethnicities, but also military veterans and people with disabilities.

Final Thoughts

The survey responses revealed that nurses have varying levels of knowledge and understanding about what is happening within nursing education, practice, and policy. There seems to be a lot of variation in what we emphasize to students and how we envision the profession. This finding is a good reminder that we need to be better at getting the word out so that everyone knows what is happening and how it affects nurses individually and collectively.

Nursing is the best profession in the world. It provides the opportunity to make a difference in the lives of others in myriad ways. Somehow, though, we nurses have been our own worst enemy by not learning from our mistakes and by introducing new ideas before truly thinking them through or attempting to permanently fix the underlying problem. I further hope we can learn from our history and accept that many of our problems have been perpetuated by our reluctance to permanently resolve them. I hope this book highlighting key aspects of important events in our history has shed light on how far we have come—unquestionably a very long way—and the tasks that lie ahead.

A SUMMARY OF KEY ISSUES

Elitism

Disunity

Not everyone can be a nurse

Broad base of knowledge

Clinical experience

Relationships

Public image

Ancillary staff

Diversity

References

Alfano, G., Anderson, H., Bitzer, M., Burnside, H., Lenbug, C. E., Campbell, R.,...Reese, V. E. M. Nursing in the decade ahead. *The American Journal of Nursing, 70*(10), 2,116–2,125.

Birnbach, N., & Lewenson, S. (Eds.). (1991). *First words: Selected addresses from the National League for Nursing 1894-1933*. New York: National League for Nursing Press.

Nightingale, F. (1860). Notes on nursing: What it is and what it is not. Retrieved from http://digital.library.upenn.edu/women/nightingale/nursing/nursing. html#III.

Index

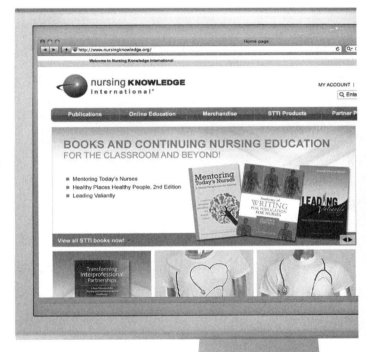

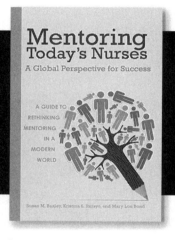
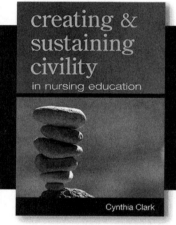
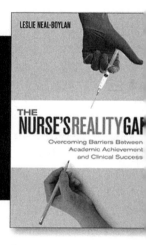

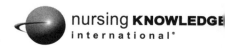